THE
Healing
Experience

THE
Healing
Experience

REMARKABLE CASES
FROM A PROFESSIONAL
HEALER

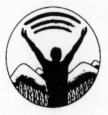

Malcolm S. Southwood

PIATKUS

© 1994 Malcolm S. Southwood

First published in 1994 by
Judy Piatkus (Publishers) Ltd
5 Windmill Street, London W1P 1HF

**The moral right of the author
has been asserted**

*A catalogue record for this
book is available from the British Library*
ISBN 0-7499-1414-9

Author photograph by Addy's of Boston, Lincs

Edited by Kelly Davis
Designed by Sue Ryall

Set in Linotron Baskerville by
PDB, London SW17
Printed and bound in Great Britain by
Bookcraft Ltd, Midsomer Norton, Avon

Life is held together
by threads of tears
which are stitched into time
to form a pattern of love
on a cloth of endeavour.

M.S.S.

My thanks to the many who have
entrusted their health and well-being to my care;
without them this book could not have
come into being.

My especial thanks to those who co-operated by
agreeing that their unique healing experience
could be written down in the hope that
it may be of help to another.

Contents

PART II The Auto Pilot: Healing the Mind and Emotions

PART III The Ejector Seat: Spiritual Healing

Foreword

I am a professional healing therapist who for over ten years has been helping people from all over the world. What follows in these pages has been learnt through the experience of treating several thousand people and keeping an open mind. It has always been my aim to cut through the dogma and the clouds of superstitious nonsense which surround much of the healing world.

I am what is termed a 'spiritual healer'. This is an awful term, for it can be interpreted in so many different and often incorrect ways. I can only write about my own experiences and beliefs and I make no claims for other healers. Healing is an individual art and, like artists, healers have their own unique style. No two artists paint alike, neither should they criticise those whose strokes of the brush are different from their own. Rather they should consider whether they could usefully learn something from another's technique.

My own philosophy is very much one of personal responsibility. I believe in a loving, creative Spirit who exists throughout all that is, guiding and assisting His many creations towards a spiritual evolution which will ensure creativity and love in place of destruction and selfishness. I believe that I am nothing without that presence of guiding love and that the only purpose of my being on this planet is what I can do for others.

I do not believe that God heals through us. Why should He? He could heal directly without our help if He chose to. Instead He has given us the power to help others if we choose. Should we use that gift in the way intended, then His great love will guide us in what we do, enabling us to give another what they need. But we must take personal responsibility for giving, and the more totally we take upon ourselves that responsibility the more of the gift, the love, there is available to give. This book has been written mainly because of the many requests I have had from clients and friends to commit to paper some of the lessons I have learnt so that others may also benefit.

So how did I get started? How does a businessman become involved in such things? At the time I was managing my own international agricultural marketing company. I also had contracts with one of the big American oil companies to manage some of their agricultural business. This work took me all over the world.

On one particular day, on my way back from London, I was held up in a line of rush hour traffic, and happened to see a notice in a window which read 'Spiritualist Church'. At the time I thought no more about it, but as the week wore on the words 'Spiritualist Church' began to haunt me. I kept asking questions about it, pestering anyone who might know what the term Spiritualist meant. I suppose I must have become quite a bore because my wife finally suggested that I go to one of their services. As she put it, 'No one here is going to get any peace until you go and find out what it's all about for yourself!' So the next weekend I attended one of their services.

I must admit that at first I thought they were all mad, especially when the minister taking the service pointed to me and said, 'You are going to be a healer for God, you are sitting in a big white aura. The work you have to do is just beginning.' Believe me, I couldn't get out of the hall fast enough. Me, a healer? Absolutely absurd. I had a wife and four children to care for, a company to run. I must have been mad even to go near the place! However, for some reason that I couldn't explain, I just couldn't stay away and each time I went I was given the same message until eventually people began to ask me to heal their headaches, knee pains and other small ailments. What was even more astonishing was the fact that I *could* and people began to come to me for help.

After a while that same voice inside which had insisted on my visiting the Spiritualist Church in the first place now told me not to visit any more. The church had served its purpose in getting me started, it said, and from now I was on my own. It might seem strange to talk about having a voice somewhere inside oneself, giving instructions, but this wasn't the first time I had had this experience. Even as a child I had heard this voice guiding, instructing and directing me and I had never had reason to think that this was anything but normal. As far as I was concerned, everyone had this protective and guiding voice. In fact there had been times in my life when it had actually spoken for me and I had listened to my own voice speaking the thoughts of another. It had got me out of more than one tricky situation. When I couldn't think of an answer I had just let this 'voice inside' speak for me.

Shortly after that, in 1979, I became very ill and spent time in the local general hospital. I remember very little about this period except that I left my body. The memory is now very vague, but I do remember going somewhere for instruction. It was like a cramming school. I suppose the medical profession would say I was hallucinating, but I wasn't. In all it lasted no more than about five days. During this time I was in an isolation ward, had two lumbar punctures and lots of tests. In the end no one ever did positively diagnose why I had suddenly collapsed in agonising pain and then drifted into some sort of semi-consciousness, but one thing was certain. The man who had gone into hospital was not the man who came out. It must have been a full twelve months before I was fully fit again and during that time I began to lose interest in my business. My whole appreciation of life and death, and all my emotional values, had changed. So had something else: my healing gift. It was now really beginning to take off and the variety of complaints which I was being asked to treat continued to increase.

Eventually I closed what was left of my agricultural business and I began to concentrate entirely on healing. I suppose I reacted in a similar way to most people when they suddenly realise they have something of value to offer. I wanted the whole world to know. My enthusiasm ran riot. The first thing I would do, I thought, would be to place adverts in the press to attract attention. At this point that little voice inside got in the way. 'Don't advertise,' it said. What rubbish, I thought. What's the point of having a gift and not using it to the full? So for the first time I ignored my guiding voice and began to work on an advertising plan.

The day after the voice had said, 'No advertising', and I had quietly, but firmly said, 'Get lost', I received a second warning not to advertise. I was expecting someone to arrive during the morning for an appointment. At the appointed time there was a knock on the door but it was not the person I was expecting. Instead there stood a vicar. I didn't know him and I must have looked surprised because he began by apologising for being there and in a somewhat embarrassed way explained that he didn't know why he had come. He had been driving along the road to an appointment when quite suddenly he had an irresistible urge to turn into our gateway and drive down our private lane to the house.

'I don't know what I'm doing here,' he said rather lamely, 'can I come in?'

He entered the room which I use for healing. I explained that unfortunately he wouldn't be able to stay for long as someone was expected. But he wasn't listening.

'What a magnificent view,' he said, looking through the bay window and across the pool immediately below it. 'What do you do?'

So I explained about my healing gift and gave him some of

my inspirational prose to read. After he had been with me about half an hour, neither of us talking, he quietly said, 'This is a beautiful place and you are not alone in it. I don't know why but I'm being forced to tell you, and I don't understand it, but under no circumstances must you advertise your gift.'

With that he got up and left and I never saw him again. Neither did I ever see the people who had booked the appointments the vicar had taken. I don't know what happened to them. This put me in a spot. I had let my company go, and with it my income, and now I couldn't advertise to attract business. But all was not lost. It wouldn't be advertising if the local doctor, with whom I was very friendly, would send me those patients that the NHS couldn't help. I went and saw him and told him what I was doing. He said he had heard and also that I had helped some of his patients already. He would suggest to those of his patients who might be interested that they also see me. I didn't see that as advertising but apparently the 'voice inside' did. I wasn't able to help a single one of the ten or twelve clients who came to me from the doctor. In fact I found that my healing gift had completely gone. I wasn't able to help anyone. So I had blown it. A chance in a lifetime to have a wonderful gift and I had thrown it away just because I thought I knew best. There was nothing for it now but to start my agricultural business up again.

About six months later, when I had given up all thoughts of healing, a lady called and asked if I would help her. She had a lot of pain from arthritis. I explained that I didn't practise healing any more, but she looked so disappointed and begged me to try just once, so how could I refuse? She came in, I put my hands over her, and 'Wow' it was back. I could feel the power surging through again and I heard a little voice inside say, 'Next time do as you are told.'

That voice guided me for a long time. Then one memorable evening, when I was giving a talk about spiritual matters to some friends, I heard my little voice say, 'It's time you began to take responsibility for these matters yourself. From now on you are on your own, learn what it is you are doing and use your own spiritual strength and love. It's been fun, but now you take over.' At this point I began to realise that there is more to healing than just putting your hands over somebody and letting another be responsible.

This book can never be more than a summary of what I have learnt about healing. It is also a very personal account and if someone, somewhere, benefits from what I write then publishing it has been worthwhile.

Finally, I feel I should explain that for ease of writing I have used the masculine term 'he' (rather than the clumsy alternatives 'he/she' or 'person') throughout the book. I hope this won't cause offence. I can assure you that the term 'he' is intended to refer to both men and women.

Malcolm S. Southwood

Introduction

There is nothing special about healers. They have not been specially chosen by God, or anybody else, because of some supernatural trait or belief. Unlike a lot of senior medical practitioners who would have us believe that they are on a plane above the common man, healers are generally ordinary people with a genuine desire to help others. Healing is a gift, though it is not granted because of a particular philosophy or to a particular individual for services rendered. It is an innate ability which many possess, though some have more ability than others. Like painting (which most of us can do to some extent), some are better at healing than others, some are better at particular aspects of healing, and we all improve dramatically the more we practise.

Some healers choose to work in groups, others singly. Some prefer to close their eyes and meditate as they heal, while others play background music. There are those who work within organised groups, such as religious organisations, while others work entirely alone. There are also a number of specialist healing groups. Some believe that you can only heal if you have completed a training course and undergone some form of initiation service or ceremony in front of your peers to prove yourself worthy of their acceptance and thereby support.

Others believe you need to have acquired belief, understanding and instruction in a particular religion or moral philosophy so that you are acceptable to God in a manner similar to themselves. At the end of the day it doesn't matter a jot what you believe, or where you go for healing instruction. An individual either does possess that extra x factor which makes him a healer or he doesn't.

So what does a healer do? Basically very little that you can see or judge. He stands behind or in front of the client, on his own or with a colleague, and passes spiritual or physical energy from or through himself to the one offering himself for treatment. As these energies flow into the client so normal health is partially or wholly restored. I say partially because healing often takes more than one treatment.

When I say a healer does very little I am not belittling him but, unlike a doctor, surgeon, psychologist or physiotherapist, there is very little apparent activity during the healing process. Unfortunately this has caused some very good healers to go rather 'over the top' in order to try and create the impression of physical or psychic activity. This is really quite unnecessary as healing is more a mental activity than a physical one. However, as I have said, healers are like artists, each one developing his own style which in no way diminishes the effect of his work. Because of the individuality of healers I will only attempt to explain what I do during my own healing sessions, as other healers may object to my particular way of working, or my interpretation of what is happening.

So just what do I do when someone comes to me for healing? We are three entities, the body, the mind and the spirit. The decision I take concerning the client depends upon whether it's a physical problem, an emotional one or a spiritual one. Basically very little can go wrong with the physical. The body is a perfectly designed piece of equipment. It is totally self regulating and self-maintaining, and only requires fuel, in the form of energy, which we get from the food we eat. Apart from genetic defects, accidents, poisoning and disease, nothing can go wrong with our machine. (Some would claim that even these four exceptions we bring upon ourselves through our attitudes and personalities.) But there is a fifth area of concern, trauma. Again, some would claim there is no such thing as coincidence, that all actions or conditions are subconsciously caused by trauma. While I would agree in some cases, I wouldn't go so far as to be categorical about it. There are shades of grey in every situation. Even so, apart from the four exceptions I have listed, I believe that most disorders are emotionally created. Healing therefore generally means helping the spirit come to terms with some situation which is troubling it so that it can work in harmony with its body. When the spirit does not work easily with the body, then the physical begins to break down.

By the time a client arrives at my door he has usually tried all the orthodox methods and reached a point where he has been told to learn to live with his problem. If any client coming for treatment has not previously seen a doctor and obviously has a medical problem then I will, of course, refuse to offer treatment unless the client first agrees to take orthodox medical advice.

Most people come to me for treatment because they are experiencing some sort of pain or discomfort. We all fear suffering, but underlying this fear is the fear of death. It's not that people are usually afraid of dying, or even becoming dead, it's more that they are afraid of the manner in which they might die and what death really means. They want to know how we get from this place to that place.

To understand this we first need to appreciate the difference between *who* we are and *what* we are. The who is the personality, that entity which in religious terminology is referred to as the spirit or soul, the part which leaves the body when we die. 'What' we are is the body, the mechanism, the means by which the spirit is able to express its ideas and emotions as personality during earthly life, the part that is left behind when we have gone. Although not made in the same way as the body, the spirit influences the functions and appearance of the body, it is using.

And, though the body should not have any influence over the spirit, weakness of spirit means that it often does. Admittedly the general direction a person takes in his life will be subject to the condition of his body and the ability of his brain. However, within these limitations, the precise direction is still the responsibility of the inhabiting spirit.

To understand what happens to us when life ends, we have to begin at the beginning, with conception. Imagine if you will that over nine months, a computerised single-seater aeroplane has been perfectly constructed for your personal use. It is a marvel of modern engineering, with its own built-in maintenance program complete with electronic surveillance system and an energy supply which is self-renewing. All it requires is someone to get aboard and fly it. That someone is you.

For a variety of reasons you have been attracted to and have entered this, as yet, untried machine. Getting into your aeroplane is the first step. For the next unknown number of years this aeroplane is your life. It is your expression of who you are. Through this flying machine, you will experience emotion and formulate your personality. And, once aboard your aeroplane, with its electro-magnetic energy fields activated, there is no way of leaving. The energy generated by the central control mechanism, the brain, cannot be switched off and the energy flowing through and around your physical body binds you into your physical shell as securely as a pilot is held by his seat belt. As long as the energy flows you are a prisoner in your aeroplane. As the body grows and develops so you learn how to control its movements — fly low, loop the loop — and how to use it as an expression of your thoughts and ideas.

Each part of the aeroplane can go wrong and will at some time need healing. The metal shell is the body. The computerised auto-pilot is the mind. Running through both is the force, the energy, that makes the plane fly, the resident spirit. Body, mind and spirit each require a different type of healing

In a sense *The Healing Experience* is both a pilot's instruction book and a repair manual. It can help you repair your own aeroplane and show you how to repair other people's.

In Part I we look at the demands made upon our machine and what happens when the fuel upon which it is dependent for smooth, efficient flying is insufficient to meet demands. In Part II we consider the part our mind, computer, plays in guiding us safely along our flight path. Finally in Part III we press the ejector button and explore the identity of spirit in aspects such as healing and reincarnation.

PART I

FLYING MANUALLY

Physical Healing

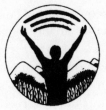

The body (our aeroplane) is one big electrically controlled machine. It has its own built-in fault finder, and if there is a breakdown in any of its circuits signals are sent out to alert the operator and action is taken to correct the fault. As with all machines it is dependent on fuel for continued, efficient flying and if for some reason our body (our aeroplane) starts to use fuel in greater quantities than it is receiving it, it will be unable to cope with our demands

Part I is about recognising and identifying faults before they become serious so that the pilot can take appropriate action before serious harm is done. A healer is a 'mechanic' who helps direct the self-maintenance system when it flashes a 'red alert'.

— 1 —

Power On

ELECTROMAGNETISM

We are all living on one gigantic magnet, the earth, which is itself controlled and powered by other magnets, especially the sun. Animals, including humans, are just tiny magnets, moving around, or being moved around, on the bigger one. Electrical stimulation within the body causes chemical reactions which lead to physical sensations and actions. One of the brain's functions is to act as the body's generator. The current it generates has to be in harmony not only with the body and all its parts but also with other electromagnetic forces, especially those produced by other people. The brain is responsible for generating a flow of electrons, a current. This somehow holds all the parts and their individual cells together as a solid form which we view as the body. The flow of electrons is more or less even, and anything which interrupts this current will cause a reaction or symptom.

Like a magnet, which has a north and south pole, the body has both negative and positive charges. A negative area of the body is a place where there is a surplus of electrons, whereas in a positive area of the body there is a scarcity of them. When electrons move away from an area, that area becomes positively charged, and the area they move to becomes negatively charged. This flow of electrons is called a current.

Positive and Negative Potentials

An electrical potential is where the conditions exist for a current but an obstruction or break in the circuit prevents the flow of electrons. The electrical potentials on the skin reflect the arrangement of the nervous system (a fact that is very well understood by acupuncturists).

From ants to humans, all life has a positive and a negative potential. In humans the head and spinal region, with its massive concentration of neurons (nerve cells), is exceptionally positive. The three main areas of greatest positive potential are the brain, the area between the shoulder blades and the base of the spinal cord. The negative areas are mainly the hands and feet and it is from their hands that healers release their energy.

Healers need to know something of this energy and how to release it from themselves to those needing it. Then their hands can act as battery terminals, linking up with those positive points on the client's body which need energy to restore the correct electromagnetic balance. The human body is one big electrical battery which can be used to charge other batteries, thus increasing their effectiveness or health.

Electromagnetic Fields

Electric fields will form around any electric charge, but they are not the same as magnetic fields. We do not really understand magnetism. All we know is that some form of identifiable and measurable matter appears within two polarities. Any flow of electrons will set up a combined electric and magnetic field around itself, producing an electromagnetic field which is stable and can be felt, measured and even photographed. This energy is sometimes called the aura and misunderstood as a spiritual energy which it most certainly is not. It is in fact the energy flowing from the cells of the body which create an electromagnetic field.

The frequency of this field is controlled by emotions originating from the mind, which is the body's computer system. As the emotions change, so will the frequency of the electromagnetic field. Its strength is dependent upon the physical health and energy reserves of the independent cells forming the body . The spirit inhabiting the body and using the mind directs the system and alters the mind's programmed responses accordingly. But all too often the spirit forgets its own part in the management of body and mind and finishes up as the passenger instead of the driver.

The whole universe is full of electromagnetic energy which can be measured as waves in electromagnetic fields. Some have suggested that this is a life force in its own right. I don't know. That it exists there is no doubt and it exists in a spectrum of wavelengths which includes radio waves, microwaves, infra-red radiation, visible light, ultra-violet radiation, x-rays, gamma rays and cosmic rays. It affects everything we do and feel. Our health depends on its balance within us and around us, and anything which affects the electromagnetic fields in our area of living is going to affect the electromagnetic fields of our bodies and therefore our health. Even the television you watch has its own electromagnetic field which will affect your personal electromagnetic field. Indeed, there is increasing evidence that very strong electromagnetic fields, like those found around power lines, can cause problems such as depression and even cancer.

THE EFFECTS OF ELECTROMAGNETIC FIELDS

Both types of fields, magnetic and electrical, can change particles as far away as outer space, even though the changes are very very slight. A body generating an electromagnetic force will therefore create a current which will affect other people close by. Everyone has their own electromagnetic field, the strength of which is dictated by their vitality and health. The frequency of the field is dictated by personality.

Harmony and Discord in Relationships

We all know people we prefer not to be with; we probably don't know why, they just make us feel uneasy. This is often because their electromagnetic field has a different frequency from our own and it will cause us distress as we try either to harmonise with it or block it out.

The effect of a frequency upon another which is different is best illustrated using a very thin layer of sand or dust on a thin metal surface. Different sounds vibrated across the surface will produce different patterns in the dust. In other words sound frequencies affect material substances. If two different sound frequencies were played on either side of the same layer of dust it would create discord. The different sound frequencies wouldn't blend and the dust wouldn't be able to take up a steady harmonious pattern. In such a situation the dust would be constantly moving and agitated.

By the same token, if a pattern formed of dust particles comes under the influence of a new sound frequency then it must either change to come into harmony with the new frequency or move away from its area of influence to prevent its pattern from breaking down. This would be a state of disease. This is exactly what happens when two people meet. Either their emotional frequencies allow companionship between them, or one will dominate the other. Alternatively, they will have to move away from each other's area of influence.

Harmony and Discord in Nature

Have you ever wondered why a robin doesn't pair up with a sparrow, or a house martin with a swallow? It's because the frequencies of their electromagnetic fields are different. Although, to us, the difference between robins and sparrows seems slight there is no way that they could pair up because the difference in their electrical fields doesn't allow for it. Don't worry if it all sounds a bit confusing. Physicists have been trying for generations to understand the mysteries of electromagnetism. Apparently not even Einstein could fathom it.

The important point to grasp is that the brain, acting as generator, controls an electric current which is produced independently by every cell in the body. Every cell is its own generator, working in harmony with the cells around it. These groups of cells collectively form organs, which work in harmony with other organs to produce electricity, all of which are controlled by the brain. If a patient undergoes a transplant operation and he is given an organ of a different electrical frequency from that of his body it is very unlikely that it will be accepted. It all depends on how closely the organ and receiving body are harmonised as to whether the two will combine.

Regeneration

In the last thirty years much evidence has been gathered to show that not only is bio-electricity a necessary energy for good health but that it is also the main stimulus in all physical regeneration. Work is being done in various countries to show that electrical currents can trigger the regeneration of bone cells as well as soft tissues. The American scientist Robert O. Becker MD has also demonstrated how it is that many of the less complex vertebrates can regenerate whole limbs through altered electrical currents. Regeneration of tissue need not be restricted to salamanders and frogs. If a child loses the end of a finger through an accident of some sort before the age of eleven, under certain circumstances the amputated part of the finger will regrow.

There was just such a case in the early 1970s at Sheffield Children's Hospital. A child who had lost the end of a finger had the wound dressed but, through a clerical mix-up, was not referred to a surgeon for further treatment. When the error was finally noted the doctor in charge noticed that the finger tip was regrowing so she merely let nature take its course and the finger regrew complete with nail. Cynthia Illingworth, the doctor concerned, started to treat other similar finger amputations in the same way and was able to show that they invariably regrew perfectly in about three months. Scientists have since measured a negative current leaving the stump.

Unfortunately most surgeons refuse to accept evidence of electrical bone regeneration or any other form of cell regeneration using electricity, preferring instead the far more costly and time-consuming yet less effective microsurgery techniques. This is despite the fact that doctors in various British hospitals have shown in the treatment of hundreds of patients that electricity will stimulate bone and tissue regeneration. Nevertheless most biologists cling to the explanation of chemical transference between cells, still believing that electricity is only a side effect of cell damage.

ELECTROMAGNETISM IN THE INDIVIDUAL

I believe that one of the brain's basic functions is to act as the body's generator — to pump, or pulse, electricity through the body. The brain somehow conducts the energy, independently created by each cell, which works in harmony with other similar cells, producing a body which functions in harmony with itself. The brain, which somehow controls the overall organisation through automatic subconscious activity is activated in turn by the inhabiting spirit. Even the spirit is very probably an electromagnetic force, whatever that is. Try holding your hands six inches from one another and you will probably feel a tingling sensation in the ends of your fingers. This is an electrical force created by two opposing negative potentials. It is this force which I refer to as energy.

Energy Obstructions

Energy is being continually pulsed through the body and as long as there is sufficient, and the flow is not interrupted, you will be physically and mentally active. The problems start when this energy is unable to get to where it is needed.

Logically it makes sense that if the pulsed electromagnetic field is interfered with, all areas beyond the point of injury (or obstruction) must in some way or other be affected.

As a healer I am able to recognise the areas of injury and so treat them with my own electromagnetic field and either improve the condition for as long as the client comes for treatment or cure the problem by removing the cause. There is nothing magical, mysterious or spiritual about this level of healing. It is just one person with a stronger electromagnetic field knowing how to use that energy to help another. I suppose the clever bit is diagnosing the cause in the first place and knowing how to use the body's electromagnetic fields to produce a cure.

Steady-state Magnetic Fields

Unorthodox healers in both India and America have made claims that by using permanent magnets they are able to cure cancer. Their results were in part confirmed when an American, Dr Kenneth Maclean, produced positive results in the 1950s and 1960s using steady-state magnetic fields to heal cancer in mice. This research is still at an early stage, but what does seem to be important is that it is the steady-state magnetic fields that hold the secret. In contrast, any pulsed or varying magnetic fields that are artificially created tend to cause stress and inhibit healing. Many healers use permanent magnets to effect improvements and, provided the steady-state magnetic field is strong enough, but at the same time not too powerful, then these methods seem to be effective.

Unfortunately there is considerable bias against electromagnetic fields among orthodox medical practitioners. Much of this has been brought on by the healers themselves who, not fully understanding what it is they are doing, make exaggerated claims about what they are achieving and what is producing the change. Guesswork and an aura of mystery are no substitute for scientific appraisal, but neither should the world of science refuse to accept what is obviously happening in the unorthodox fields just because they can't fit it into their existing knowledge without abandoning some long-treasured theory.

THE EFFECTS OF RADIO WAVES

At one stage in my career I was involved with experimental work using radio waves to stimulate growth in plants. We did this in many ways, one of which was to pass radio waves through water in which we had immersed seeds. We were able to demonstrate that seeds with low germination and vitality levels could be invigorated with life after just twenty minutes' treatment, and if we then used the treated water on other plants those plants grew faster and stronger than plants given untreated water. We also passed radio waves through a strip of ground and all the plants along the treated line responded with faster growth. Something similar can be seen where any high-voltage power line runs across farming land. Our results became more bizarre when we placed fertilised chicken's eggs in water through which radio waves were being transmitted. The eggs hatched up to 20 per cent faster than untreated eggs but the abnormalities in the chicks were horrendous and we didn't continue with this side of our work. In one test I carried out (and in no way could it be described as a controlled experiment) I drank water which had had radio waves passed through it at one particular frequency. After about a week I noticed that I was becoming increasingly intolerant and friends assured me that I was exhibiting all the signs of a personality change. The same reaction was observed in animals which had access to similarly treated water. We all quickly returned to normal behaviour patterns when we again drank normal water. But as the body is 70 per cent fluid, we must consider ourselves at risk when in too close a proximity to radio waves.

Is the increase in radio waves in our atmosphere one of the reasons for the growing intolerance in society today? I don't know, though one can't help wondering about the long term effect on people who constantly use head-phones to listen to music. Perhaps if they had been privy to some of the research I have seen they wouldn't be quite so keen on passing radio waves through their brains. Radio waves can adversely affect our health and electrical pollution is probably just as great a threat to the environment as chemical pollution. Anything which interferes with the regular flow of electrical current through the body is bound to cause problems. As Dr Becker puts it in his excellent book, *The Body Electric*:

> *All life pulsates in time to the earth and our artificial fields cause abnormal reactions in all organisms ... What will we do if the incidence of deformed children rises to 50%, if the cancer rate climbs to 75%. Will we be able to pull the plug?*

— 2 —

Circuit Breakers

Electricity pulsing through the body stimulates cell division. If for some reason the pulsed electrical current is interfered with, then the cells it stimulates will be adversely affected. There is some work being done by bioelectricians which goes a long way to confirm this, and my own healing experience also supports it.

—— CANCER AND BACK INJURIES ——

A few years ago a man who had liver cancer came to see me. He had been told that, short of a liver transplant, there was no way he would survive. At the time he was being treated at a London hospital, and as a liver transplant was out of the question his future seemed very bleak. He wasn't very old, somewhere in his early forties. His condition had been diagnosed two or three years earlier and he had been slowly deteriorating ever since. There had been no treatment and he had stopped work almost as soon as the condition was diagnosed. Like most others, he came to see me because there was really nowhere else to go.

This man was the first of several similar cases in which I have found that the cause of the problem was an undetected back injury. In his working days he had been a motor mechanic and had somehow damaged the lumbar region of his spine. Apart from the occasional ache the problem had seemed to clear up, and anyway he now had liver cancer, making his back injury seem very unimportant. However I was not so sure, especially as I was picking up his spinal injury as pain in my spine.

Having located the position in his damaged spine through which the electricity passes to control liver functions I concluded that the nerves must have been damaged at this point and that this was why his liver had started to produce malignant cells. I therefore disregarded his liver and concentrated on his injured back. For several weeks he had terrible backache after each healing session. This was because the healing was affecting the muscle tension around the vertebra, but slowly and surely the liver began to improve until it had returned to normal.

That was four and a half years ago and the specialists are still trying to decide what it was that could have caused such a dramatic recovery. They will not accept that a healer with no medical knowledge could have known something or reversed something which was beyond them. Incidentally this man was still very healthy and at work as of the spring of 1994.

I have used exactly the same method to help with cancer of the stomach and lungs. And I am now of the firm belief that many cancers are caused by no more than an interference in the normal flow of electrical currents along the nerves. I have even helped a patient who came to me with asthma by treating his back. At the beginning of treatment he was on high doses of steroids and hadn't been able to work for two years. Again it became evident that he had suffered a back injury, this time right at the base of his spine. I located this by picking up the pain in my own spine (which is something I am able to do when I harmonise with a patient). The patient hadn't thought to tell me about it, believing that it wasn't important.

When I questioned him he explained that he had had an accident at work some six or seven years earlier. His asthma had started about six months after his accident. When he stopped to consider the implications of what I was suggesting he also remembered that his worst asthma attack had occurred shortly after he hurt his back a second time.

After his first treatment he began to improve dramatically and it wasn't many weeks before the asthma symptoms had more or less disappeared and, with his doctor's approval, he began to reduce his steroids. After four weeks he had taken up singing again, a hobby which he had had to give up. By this time he had reduced his steroids to a fifth of the original dose. After four months he stopped taking his steroid tablets and his asthma has not returned since.

And it doesn't stop there. I have had quite spectacular results for a whole series of complaints where there has been a problem with the spine and the injury doesn't have to be a major one.

PHYSICAL PAIN

Pain, through injury or stress, must be one of the most common problems I have to deal with. Taken together, muscular pain and backache account for the greater part of all my consultations. The majority of people have already been to their local doctor and may have been referred to clinics or hospitals for specialist treatment, but the pain persists in spite of all the drugs used to cure it. So, what is pain? It comes in so many forms based on where it is, what's causing it, whether it's physical or emotional, and the individual's ability to control it.

Pain is caused by damage to body tissue. The damaged cells discharge chemicals called prostaglandins. These chemicals act on the nerve endings so that an electrical current is passed along the sensor nerves to the brain. There is a bit more to it than that, but basically the brain accepts this signal and returns an electrical current to the point of injury which stimulates tissue repair. This electrical stimulation causes the cells to multiply. However, until the process is complete, the pain remains, as the prostaglandins continue to be released to ensure continued electrical stimulation and healing.

———————— *TRAPPED NERVES* ————————

Headaches are often caused by a build-up of current which is unable to flow, due to a break or blockage somewhere in the circuit. I have helped many migraine sufferers simply by identifying an injury in a nerve which is preventing the current discharging from the brain. The current builds up and eventually overloads the system; the surplus is then burnt off as pain, in the form of a migraine. Anything which causes excess energy in the body can produce a headache or migraine if there is a block on that nerve line. The block acts like a switch which is permanently in the 'off' position and the overloaded circuit then 'blows a fuse'. This is not to say all migraines are due to trapped nerves but in my experience some of them are.

A typical example was a man in his late forties who had been having severe migraines on a regular basis for over two years. He came to me with the beginnings of a migraine which made finding the problem much easier. When I put both hands over his head the pain became much worse (as you would expect because I was adding to the energy in the overloaded circuits). I then put my left hand on his wrist while keeping my right hand above his head. The effect was dramatic. It was as if I had switched something off. All his migraine pain ceased immediately, not slowly, or after a second or two, but instantly. I then took my hand off his wrist and put it back over his head and 'pow', the pain returned, just as quickly as it had stopped. I repeated the process several times and each time I got the same dramatic and immediate effect, from pain to no pain, and back again.

So somewhere between the brain and the wrist there was a trapped nerve. When I put my hands over his head and wrist I was obviously bypassing the block and completing the circuit.

On questioning him, he told me that when he was about five he had broken his elbow, but it obviously couldn't be that as the migraines had only started some two years previously. After further questioning he remembered an accident at work when he had fallen heavily on his shoulder about two and a half years earlier. So this had to be it. The fall had somehow caused a nerve to become trapped in the shoulder.

Being a big strong man, the occasional ache or pain hadn't bothered him and anyway the migraines were far more worrying. On its own the trapped nerve in his shoulder probably wouldn't have caused any problems but if the old elbow injury was blocking the same nerve it was very probable that the double damage was creating too much resistance in the electrical circuit. I massaged and gave healing to his shoulder for half an hour and apart from a couple of times he hasn't had another migraine in over four years.

— *PAIN AND ELECTROMAGNETIC FIELDS* —

If you place a strong enough magnetic field at right angles to the flow of an electrical current it interrupts the flow of electricity and the pain ceases. This has proved to be just as effective as drug-induced pain control in many situations. And this is basically what a healer with a sufficiently strong electromagnetic field of his own does when he puts his hands over an injury. But if he happens to place his hands in line with the patient's own flow of current he can actually increase the level of pain. It took me quite a while to work this out.

Effective healing is not just putting your hands in any position, it's knowing where to place them, how close to place them and remembering that the aim is not just to stop pain but to effect healing. To achieve this, the current to the site of injury needs to be increased to speed up the healing process, without letting the increased current find its way back to the brain. As you will appreciate this calls for a little extra understanding of

the principles of electromagnetism in relation to brain stimulation and increased cell activity. After a healer has given his
treatment, the pain at the site of injury will often increase for
one to three days, after which it should disappear completely.
What happens is that while the healer is giving his 'hands on'
treatment he effectively stops electrical flow, while increasing
potential at the injury site. When he removes his hands the flow
pattern returns to normal. As the extra electrical potential at
the injury eventually registers with the brain so the pain
perceived is correspondingly increased, but the healing effect is
positive. It's surprising just how effectively wounds will heal
after receiving a 'hands on' treatment.

I think the pain of any injury is probably caused by the
stimulation of extra electrical activity at the site of injury. Pain
does not always occur at the moment of injury. It often follows
seconds or even hours later. Pain is the extra electrical activity
at the nerve ends which causes cell multiplication in order to
produce new tissue.

Direct currents within the central nervous system regulate
the sensitivity of the nerve cells in several ways: by changing the
amount of the current; by reversing its polarity; and by
changing its frequency. All these things are controlled by the
subconscious and they can all be influenced by a good healer
with a strong electromagnetic field. Many healers switch in to
the patient's condition by reacting to the patient's area of injury.
They then adjust their own electromagnetic field to that
required by the patient, so boosting the patient's own healing
abilities.

As I have already stated, a sufficiently strong magnetic field
at right angles to a current magnetically stops the flow and this
has been proved to be just as effective as chemical anaesthesia.
If you pass a current through the brain from front to back it will
cancel out the normal current and cause unconsciousness.

It is well known that brain waves vary with changes in
consciousness. A healer can adjust these brain wave cycles to
the ideal level of eight to fourteen a second (which are called

alpha waves) by placing his hands over the patient's head. This puts the person into the state we experience just before waking or sleeping, and this is very possibly how hypnosis works.

If a healer reduces the current in the brain to ten cycles per second his patient will be totally relaxed, yet not asleep. This is exactly the effect that most people report when visiting a healer. Fortunately most healers say nothing while their patients are in this state, just allowing them to enjoy the relaxation.

A healer can use his own energies to increase his patient's direct current in the area of the injury. Increasing the current increases cell repair activity at the site of the injury.

PAIN AND MUSCLES

If the bioelectricity in a body is reduced, muscles tighten. Look at what happens to a corpse. As soon as life is extinguished it begins to stiffen. Furthermore, as the current is reduced, so is the electromagnetic field. And as the electromagnetic field weakens, so gravitational effect increases and the body becomes heavier.

It is this which causes the limbs of those affected by a stroke to feel heavy. The electrical current to the limb is blocked, due to nerve damage in the brain. Without current there is no electromagnetic field around the affected limb, and because an electromagnetic field opposes gravitational pull the limb feels heavier than an unaffected limb. This is what is meant by a 'dead weight'. A 75 kg body will be easily moved if there is life in it, but the moment life ceases it becomes extraordinarily heavy (ask any nurse), although it's been proved that the body actually loses a few ounces at death.

It is easier to lift something if you take hold of it for a few minutes beforehand, rather than trying to lift it immediately. This is quite simply because your energy has had time to flow through and around the object. It is always easier to lift something which is included in your own electromagnetic field. Bioelectricity is like a bubble or an aura which you travel in for ease and comfort. If for any reason your energy levels drop, your electromagnetic field will drop and the anti-gravity bubble which is transporting you over the earth's magnetic surface will begin to weaken. Your ability to move will decrease relative to the weakening of your bubble.

On any sunny day we all feel brighter and more relaxed, whereas on cold, sunless days we tend to feel stiffer. The colder the day, the more energy we utilise to keep warm. And the more energy we utilise but don't replace, the weaker our electromagnetic field becomes and the stiffer we feel. This is not so extraordinary when you bear in mind that reptiles need the sun's energy to become active. They don't have the capacity to create energy themselves, or store it in sufficient quantities to keep them mobile. We are not quite so dependent on the sun, though some people are dramatically affected by any lack of sunlight.

Many clients come to me with stiff muscles and most of them are utilising more energy than they are absorbing. Often the situation is made worse when the sufferer is eating large quantities of red meat. Meat is muscle and have you ever considered the strength in the muscles of a cow? When you eat beef you are taking in the chemicals built into the muscle fibres which cause them to contract. When taken into your system these chemicals are added to your own, thus adding to your muscle strength. That's why boxers and weight-lifters eat a lot of beef. It builds muscle. That is fine provided the muscles relax when you want them to. But problems arise if you are unable to increase your bioelectricity to cope with the extra muscle strength. If you don't your muscles won't relax properly, which causes endless problems.

Another problem with beef, I believe, is that when an animal is slaughtered it is in a state of shock. Anyone who has visited a slaughterhouse will vouch for this. Cows are very sensitive animals and very prone to fear. Fear triggers the release of adrenalin into the muscle system to allow for faster reaction and greater contraction of the muscles. Nothing is done or can be done, to remove this added adrenalin from the carcase. I presume, therefore, that it must remain in the meat. This increases the diner's adrenalin level, causing all his muscles to stiffen. It would be interesting to see some work done on this aspect of nutrition. Anyone with rheumatoid arthritis will know that eating beef causes extra pain. I have one patient who only has to have a beef sandwich to be aware of extra pain a few hours later. It stands to reason that if your muscles are stronger, or tighter, they will cause the joints to tighten. Without muscles you wouldn't have stiff joints; it is opposing muscle contraction which causes joint movement. The greater the total overall muscle tension, the more difficult it becomes to move the joints and as the joints tighten because of over-tight muscles so overall movement becomes slower, more difficult and more painful.

MUSCLES AND BONES

Nearly all back pain which I treat is due to excessive muscle tension. In all the years I've been treating patients who have come to me complaining that they have a disc out only twice have I had to send them on to a chiropractor or osteopath. In most cases I just relax the muscles and the disc slips back on its own. Let's take a typical example.

A patient bends or twists to pick something up. As the muscles pulling him up contract, so the opposing muscles relax, allowing the body to straighten. If the opposing muscles don't relax, something has to give and usually it's the contracting muscle. This results in a lot of pain and takes quite a while to heal. The bones to which they are attached are sometimes also pulled very slightly out of position. If the vertebrae are involved then pulling them out of alignment with each other causes the disc to move. You can put that disc back as often as you like, but it won't stop there until the muscles relax, allowing the bones to re-align.

Wherever you get over-tense muscles you will get stiffness and pain. It matters not whether it's in the back, the shoulders or the legs; if the muscles are too tight for easy joint movement you will have pain. Furthermore if the joints are too tight they will begin to wear out (especially hip joints, eventually leading to hip replacements). Stress, being a condition of 'more energy used than consumed', always results in stiff muscles accompanied by pain, especially in the shoulder area. All a competent healer has to do is place his hands over or near the nearest positive potential. At no time is any manipulation necessary or recommended. Manipulation should be carried out by qualified physiotherapists only and if it is necessary the healer should send the client to see a doctor. Let me give a few classic examples of muscular pain.

The first involves a young woman of twenty-three. Someone had run into the back of her car three years earlier. As a result of the accident she had suffered a whiplash injury which was the basis of an insurance claim. Three years later, the insurance company was still arguing about the seriousness of the injury. They wanted her to see another specialist who was prepared to do a very delicate and potentially risky operation on her neck which had become very stiff. Rather than have an operation, she came to me to see what could be done. She was wearing a surgical collar to prevent head movement, having been told that any head movement would result in more damage. She was also in constant pain.

I sat her in an upright chair and asked her to remove the surgical collar she was wearing. I then asked her to close her eyes which makes relaxing easier. I put my fingers on either side of her neck. After about five minutes she began to sob, uncontrollably at first, as the trauma released itself. About five minutes after this her head began to move involuntarily and soon it was shaking up and down and rolling from side to side. This continued for about twenty minutes. At the end of the twenty minutes I took my hands away, let her rest for a minute or so and then asked her to move her head. There was absolutely no restriction in her movements. All her pain had gone and she has had no further problem since.

I was asked to write a note for the insurance company and doctor. Briefly my explanation was that at the time of the accident shock-waves had travelled through her body and been absorbed by the neck muscles. This latent energy had not been released. Furthermore the young woman had been reduced to a state of severe shock which had not been treated so that the system of muscles around her neck and shoulders had become locked. This was because of the unreleased energy within the muscles and also because of the untreated shock which, in other circumstances, would probably have passed in a month or so and eased the problem. She subsequently lost her claim against the insurance company but that didn't seem to worry her too much.

I have had several of these sort of situations to deal with. I also get quite a number of patients asking for help with a condition called spondulosis. This is a tightening of the muscles around the vertebra, causing them to become worn. Some are beyond my help, though most receive either complete or partial cure. As always, I need to begin by identifying the cause of the stress. Those I usually fail to help are the more elderly people. Personally I don't believe there is any reason why anyone should suffer spondulosis if it is treated early enough. Any treatment which relaxes muscles will cure the condition, though it will not mend worn or damaged bone. However, this condition does need to be treated early and the cause identified or the symptoms will return. Although the symptoms show in the joints, the problem is the overtight muscles.

Let's face it. Apart from disease, not a lot can go wrong with the bones. A skeleton without muscle wrapped around it isn't going to wear, as the joints will be very free and loose. It's only when muscles tighten around the bones that problems start. It really is essential that muscle tension is regularly checked. Bone wear can often be directly attributed to over-tensed muscles which are tight because of a bioelectrical system which is not up to strength. Sometimes this is the result of shock, emotional pressure or other forms of stress, all of which utilise energy.

It would be a big step forward in medicine and preventative health care if some means could be found of measuring and quantifying the human electromagnetic field, or even muscle tension. It sometimes takes physiotherapists months to relax the muscles sufficiently to see improvement. And unless they have done something to increase the bioelectrical potential of the patient, and considered action to deal with the stress which originally caused it, then conventional means are unlikely to result in permanent success. To anyone with the painful and restricting condition of spondulosis I would say go and see a registered healer, not for manipulation, but for ordinary healing. From a healer's point of view it really is one of the easier problems to deal with.

One situation I remember, involving muscle problems, concerned a fourteen-year-old boy. The boy had developed a very bad limp and it had been suggested that he have an operation to correct the problem.

His father, who came with him, explained that the problem was something to do with the bones or tendons of his foot. I naturally accepted this explanation of the problem and began by looking for a changed electrical potential in the foot. But try as I might I couldn't find one, and I became more and more convinced that the problem was not in the foot at all but in the hip. But, with father watching my every move and having been so sure about where the problem was, I ignored my own feelings and continued trying to treat the lad's foot.

After about fifteen minutes of wasted time when there hadn't been any result from what I was doing, I came to my senses and, ignoring what father had told me, turned my attention to the boy's hip. Immediately, I got a reaction and his leg began to twist and turn as the healing energy found its way to the problem. The fault lay, not in the foot, but in a muscle somewhere in the thigh which had gone into spasm, a sort of permanent cramp. It took about ten minutes to free the muscle, after which he got up and walked around the room perfectly, with no signs of a limp at all. He came again the following week just in case the problem had returned, as it sometimes does in this type of situation, but he was still perfectly free and as far as I know never had any more difficulty.

Cramp-type symptoms are responsible for a lot of backache. It's not at all unusual to have a pain in one hip when the cause of the problem is in the other. Let's say through strain, particularly such as standing on a ladder or chair and reaching up on one leg, the muscles on, say, the left side become strained. Hours later they will usually go into a sort of cramp but without pain. At best the muscle doesn't relax totally after the effort or strain put on it. Because the muscles in the left leg are now in a semi-contracted state they pull the joints tighter together.

This contraction of the muscles actually shortens the affected leg, usually only by about 1 or 2 centimetres. With the left leg now being that little bit shorter, the right leg has to carry more weight, both standing and walking. Unless both legs are of equal length there is bound to be unequal pressure. This will be exerted on the hip of the longer side and that is where the pain begins to show. Eventually this unequal pressure will cause the right hip to wear and the back to ache, though usually the back aches long before the hip is affected.

Any treatment is therefore needed on the left hip. It's a waste of time to treat the pain in the right side because that is just a symptom. The cause of the discomfort is in the left side even though there are no symptoms in that area. Only a few weeks ago I had a man call who had had pain in his left hip and back for nearly twenty years. The trouble was exactly as described above, and after treating his right leg for two weeks his pain has totally gone. Again, I make the point that no amount of drugs, massage, or other treatment for backache on the painful side will be of any benefit until the tension on the seemingly good side has been attended to.

On one occasion a young man came to see me with a back and hip pain on his left side. He was a groom working for a racing stable. Some years earlier he had had a riding accident and broken a bone in his right leg which was now about 2 centimetres shorter than his left leg. I decided that the pain he was getting in his left hip was a direct result of the right leg being that bit shorter and causing extra pressure to be extended up the left side of his body. If he had attempted to walk evenly he would have spent all his life going around in circles. I sat him down, took the weight of his right leg in my hands by holding his foot and let the healing energy pass up through his muscles. Within a few minutes his leg was involuntarily twisting and jumping. After about fifteen minutes we compared the length of his legs and they were now both the same. When he stood up he had a few problems coordinating at first, while his brain readjusted to the new walking position, but that soon sorted itself out.

He returned the following week for a check-up. The pain in the left side had gone and he said that he had had to lengthen his stirrup for the right leg by 2.5 centimetres. Apparently he had ridden with a shorter stirrup on the one side ever since his accident. His only complaint was that on the evening of the day he visited me he had gone to his local pub for a game of darts and found it almost impossible to hit the board because his stance had been so improved by the healing. I have treated others with similar problems and the results are always painless, quick and permanent.

Before moving off the association between over-tight muscles and pain I'll give another example. I've changed the name, as always, though this case is well known.

It had been ten-year-old Sally's dream to win the 1990 summer riding events at the local branch of the Pony Club. She was understandably devastated when the doctors explained to her that the pain she was having in her knees was a condition called Osgood-Schlatter's disease. It usually appears in children approaching puberty and is caused by an excess of bone growth in the joints around the knee. This results in loss of movement, intense pain and eventually splintering of the bone forming the joint. It is thought to be incurable but Sally was told she would grow out of it as she matured towards adulthood. The condition tends to appear in children who take part in a sport.

Sally's problem started in June 1990 and made even walking difficult. The only suggestion the doctor could give was to put her leg into plaster to restrict movement. In October 1990, Sally's parents brought her to me. She had regular weekly sessions which brought almost immediate relief from the pain and swelling in the affected joints. By Christmas of that year she was virtually back to normal and totally free of pain. In May of the following year, 1991, Sally went on to receive bronze and silver awards for swimming, she came second in a Pony Club competition for both dressage and show jumping, and first in an open junior competition that year. Not bad for a girl who was told she wouldn't be able to walk properly until she was sixteen.

So, what was the problem? And what cured it? Most people fail to understand that bones grow but muscles don't. Muscles are stretched by the growing bones and this causes new muscle fibres to grow, thus maintaining the correct muscle tension in relation to the bones. Some children have strong muscles and a tendency for the tension in their muscles to be above average for their age. When these children are encouraged to participate in sports, particularly those requiring strength, the muscles become too strong in relation to the bones they are supporting. This means that the growing bones cannot stretch the muscles, which causes the bones to start growing into each other and forces them out of position.

Sally had been riding big horses since she was a little girl. This had caused her leg and thigh muscles to over-develop. In fact she had very strong arm, leg and thigh muscles. All very necessary if you going to ride and control a powerful horse, but not very helpful to a growing bone which needs to stretch the muscles attached to it, so it can grow further. Sally's bones were just not strong enough to stretch the muscles; instead, the muscles held the bones tight causing bone to grow into bone until eventually the joints of her knees were forced out of shape and the bones began to grow through the muscle. Healing relaxed Sally's muscles to the extent that the growing bones were able to move back into place.

There are such things as 'growing pains', as this particular incident graphically illustrates. I have a lot of young people who come for treatment, their only problem being over-developed muscles. These are just the sort of situations in which healing can prove very successful. Drug therapy, surgery and the like are not the answer to a problem which requires muscle relaxation. I'm afraid steroids are also often used as a muscle relaxant. I do wish that more doctors would recommend healing therapy first. It might just save everyone a lot of pain and misery.

The older the sufferer of this sort of condition, the more difficult it is to overcome it. Obviously, as we age, so the muscle strength and bone positioning become more permanent. If you have a child with muscle problems, and conventional treatment is not helping, ask your doctor to recommend a qualified experienced healer. Remember, healing therapy does not involve the use of manipulation and registered healers will not attempt it unless they are qualified to do so.

——————— *ENERGY AND WATER* ———————

One form of exercise which can lead to muscle or bone pain is swimming. I know all the arguments about it being a relaxing way of exercising and think it's one of the best and safest sports you can do. But for anyone not physically fit or suffering from rheumatism, depression and other similar conditions I would not recommend it. In fact I go so far as to instruct some of the people I'm treating not to go swimming until I say they can.

The reason behind this is quite simple. As I keep explaining, one of the main causes of bone or muscle pain is that over-tensed muscles do not allow freedom of movement between the joints. This is often due to low energy, low levels of current in the body and a correspondingly low bioelectrical field. Water and electricity don't mix. So why do people go swimming when their energy levels are already below what is required for a relaxed body?

Whatever your energy was before, once in the pool your bioelectricity will be conducted through the water, to be expelled into the air above it. Swimmers get cramp for this very reason. The very fit will be able to withstand the energy loss for longer than those with lower reserves, but eventually all swimmers succumb to fatigue and cramp if they stay in the water long enough. So if you go for a swim you will lose energy.

I'm not referring to the energy you will burn up with the effort of swimming. This loss is to be expected, and if you leave the water before your reserves have been unduly leached out by the water all will be well. But if you enter the water with your reserves of energy already low, your problems are likely to become worse. I know that it is sometimes recommended that people who suffer from arthritis should take up swimming, but I believe anyone who has a low energy level to start with will only aggravate their problem by swimming.

I know all the arguments about how much better they feel while they are swimming. Of course they do. For a short while the skeletal frame is not having to support any weight, and this relieves pain. Also, as I pointed out earlier, pain is an indication of excess energy flowing into an area to cause a healing activity. Swimming leaches out the energy, so relieving the pain. But it later aggravates the problem, unless the sufferer is very fit and energetic to start with. If you believe that swimming is helping you, good, stay with it. If it's not, stay out of the water and certainly don't go within three days of seeing a healer or you will dilute his work (please excuse the pun).

This is why fish are cold-blooded. They can't store bioelectricity. They have electric current, but not an electro-magnetic field. It's because water conducts electricity so efficiently that it releases it to the atmosphere. This is why we feel relaxed when we sit beside a river or pool. We absorb the energy that the river is discharging. Maybe this is why people get more arthritis in damp climates. A damp atmosphere may affect our bioelectric field by conducting the electromagnetic energy to a greater area, causing the muscles to tighten and joints to suffer.

REFERRED PAIN

If you have pain anywhere do not necessarily expect the cause to be in the same place. It doesn't always follow. If ever I needed proof of this it came with a man who had had backache for many years. His work involved a lot of driving and his back pain had become so severe, especially while he was driving, that he was seriously thinking of giving it all up. He had had all the usual treatments, pain-killers, physiotherapy, massage, and over the years he had spent a small fortune on seeing various private therapists and specialists.

At last he arrived at my door. I put my hands over his lower back, over his hips and along the full length of his spine and could find no problems whatsoever. Then I checked his legs, ankles and down to his feet. As I ran my hand over the bridge of his right foot I felt a resistance to my electromagnetic field (aura). So I just lightly pressed the top of his foot. The effect was instant and dramatic.

'Quickly!' he shouted. 'Never mind my foot, the pain has come into my back. It's there now, it's terrible.'

So I took my finger off his foot to go to his back and the pain began to ease. Then I had my answer. 'Have you ever twisted your ankle?' I asked.

'About five years ago, but what has that got to do with it?'

'Tell me what happened,' I continued.

'Well, I was walking down some steps and the right ankle cobbled over and it hurt like hell for about a week, but then it soon cleared up. Why?'

I then asked him when he had first experienced his backache and he told me about four and a half years ago (which was about six months after he twisted his ankle). I then explained that when he had twisted his ankle he had somehow exposed a nerve in the top of his foot. How this happened I didn't know. But after that every time something touched that particular nerve a pain registered in his back.

I had no idea why the pain should be referred to his back and I had even less idea how to treat it, but I suggested that in future he wore a type of shoe which doesn't have a lace tie. Then when he's driving and wants to ease his foot up off the accelerator there won't be any pressure from the laces to cut across the top of his foot and affect the nerve. This was one of those cases I couldn't cure but could help in showing how to avoid the pain.

Not all symptoms are what they seem to be and the next case is typical of what I mean. In the twelve years I've been healing I've had a few of these sorts of oddities and they do keep you on your toes.

A man came to me with a heart and breathing problem. He would get up feeling well enough but as soon as he went outside he would begin to get chest cramp, his lungs would seize up and leave him gasping for air, and the pain in his chest was indescribable. The doctors had examined him thoroughly and could find no cause for his problems. He worked in a stuffy factory, and on those occasions that he had managed to get to work breathing difficulties soon forced him to return home. It was the same in the evening. He was all right as long as he stayed inside the house but the moment he went out into the cold air, down he went.

This had been going on for six months before he came to see me. I listened to his story and then went into the usual healing position which is standing behind and over the patient. As my healing energies began to work he started to get very hot (he obviously wasn't short of energy). But the hotter he got, the more effective his anti-perspirant became, and its perfume became stifling. It was a very strongly scented one, and the longer the healing went on the stronger the perfume and its fumes became, until I could stand it no longer.

'How long have you been using this anti-perspirant?' I asked.

'That's a funny question,' he said 'About six months I suppose. Why?'

'Do you always spray it on in the bathroom?'

'Yes.'

'Do you use plenty of it, perhaps twice a day?'

'I suppose so, but what has that got to do with my chest?'

'I don't know what it does to your chest,' I said, 'but in ten minutes the fumes of it are almost choking me. If you are spraying this stuff in a small, air-tight bathroom I suspect that you are breathing the stuff in. As an antiperspirant it has a drying factor in it. And I expect it's drying your lungs out, so that when you go outside and breathe in the cold air your lungs tighten up. You are supposed to put the antiperspirant under your armpits, not down your lungs. I suggest you stop using it for a week or two, especially as it's the same six months that you've been having this problem.'

He came to see me once more, two weeks later, his problem gone.

I had a similar case with a lady who used lots of hair lacquer every morning to hold her hair in place. She also sprayed the stuff on to her hair in a small room so that she was bound to finish up breathing it in. The only facts the doctors had been given were that she was feeling faint, dizzy and having breathing problems. No amount of drugs were going to help in this case. Once I had pointed out what she was doing and stopped her using the hair lacquer, her health returned.

Healing also means being observant and using some intuition and a lot of common sense.

— 3 —

Maintenance

Most people in the world today are suffering from some form of physical stress, which means that they are utilising more energy than they are absorbing or creating. There are several early and obvious symptoms, though it would seem that few of them are recognised by the general public until it is too late. Here is a quick checklist:

- Difficulty sleeping
- Stiff limbs or even cramp
- Difficulty moving around
- Feeling tired
- Difficulty remembering things
- Feeling cold, especially feet and hands
- Difficulty with comprehension, e.g. becoming confused if reading a long passage or forgetting the beginning before reaching the end
- Difficulty making decisions
- Having a sweet tooth
- And many more.

If a client came to me with some of these symptoms I would consider that he might be lacking the fuel of life, energy, and without energy his engine, his body, will not function. Most of the people who come to see me are burning up more energy than they are taking in, if for no other reason than that they are worried.

A good healer with an abundance of surplus energy will pass that surplus to his patient who will begin to feel relaxed and even tired. There may even be a few tears. (One of the most necessary items in my treatment room is a box of tissues.) A person under stress is like a car with a flat battery — mechanically sound but without recharging they can't get going. Nothing lights up any more. Once the battery is topped up and the engine is running again it very quickly recharges from its own efforts.

TENSE MUSCLES

One of the first signs of energy loss is a tightening of the muscles. For the purpose of explaining the importance of bioelectricity, especially as a healing force, I am omitting all reference to the part played by chemicals, oxygen etc. Take, for example, athletes who have finished a race and used up all their surplus energy. It's not unusual to see them go down with cramp. This, I believe, is due to insufficient energy pulsing through the muscles to keep them relaxed.

Most of us are not athletes and don't tend to experience cramp unless our energy supply runs very low. It's more common for muscles just to tighten. We usually notice this first across the shoulders, down the back and then at later stages down the arms and legs. Electromagnetic energy flows in waves through the body. How this is caused I don't know but as a healer I can feel my energy flowing through me and I have no doubt that it is being pulsed. Every muscle in the body is tightening, relaxing, tightening, relaxing, at different speeds as energy passes through them.

The heart is the obvious example with its regular beat. This pumping action of grip, release, is present in every muscle and helps to keep the body toned up. Furthermore, it helps to keep the blood moving through the body. There is no way a heart, unaided, can pump blood through capillaries in your toes without the help of muscle action. Should the muscles start to tighten because of low energy, there's a more than even chance that your blood pressure will start to rise. Not only will the heart be pumping without any help from the muscles, but the tightening muscles will be putting pressure on the arteries and veins running through them. Stiffening muscles causing high blood pressure often indicate low energy or, if you prefer the name by which it is more commonly known, stress. Also, as we have already seen, when muscles tighten they pull bones closer together, causing stiff joints which rub and wear against each other.

How your healer treats you will depend on his own technique. I work on the basis that if the problem is above the waist I put my hands over the head, either side of the neck or on the shoulder. If the problem is mainly below the waist I put my hands in the middle of the lower back. The effect can be quite dramatic, especially with problems such as sciatica. I take hold of the ankles if there is a subconscious barrier and usually within a few minutes the muscles are twitching and the legs jumping around as the over-tight limbs loosen up. Most cases of lower backache and sciatica are nothing more than a form of cramp anyway. As the energy passes from healer to client so the client will begin to feel warmer. I should point out that most people can boost their own energy levels without ever going to a healer and many can prevent themselves from sliding down into stress or depression if they take action to maintain a healthy bioelectrical field.

It is not always possible for the people in stressful situations to change the situation which is causing the stress or to remove themselves from it. That only leaves one alternative, to increase the levels of energy consumed to meet physical requirements. More of this when we have discussed all the symptoms.

FEELING COLD

Another symptom of low energy is a general feeling of cold, particularly cold feet. I never cease to be surprised when people tell me that the reason they suffer from cold feet is because of poor circulation. Are they saying that the blood isn't getting to the feet, that it's getting to the ankles but then suddenly and inexplicably flowing more slowly, only to speed up again as it enters the legs? To say that continual cold feet are due to poor circulation is totally illogical. If blood wasn't getting to the feet, then other, greater problems would soon become apparent.

It isn't only blood which maintains body temperature. It's electrical current. Take an electric light. When you switch it on, the bulb heats up; when you switch it off, it goes cold. Electricity or energy flowing around the body and overcoming resistance creates heat, helping to maintain body temperature. If your energy is low your body temperature will also be low, especially in the feet which are furthest removed from the brain, or generator.

I have shown time and time again that cold feet are usually directly associated with low levels of energy or some other condition affecting the body's energy levels. As the condition worsens so the feeling of cold spreads through the whole body.

INSOMNIA

Another symptom that can sometimes be directly related to low energy is insomnia. As I have already said, we need energy to keep the muscles relaxed, the heart beating, the lungs pumping and so on. But what happens when we go to sleep and our brain wave activity, electrical energy, is virtually switched off ? In order to accommodate sleep, which is essential for brain rest, the body needs to hold potential energy in reserve. It holds it in the form of glucose — in the liver and elsewhere.

If our muscles don't have the required reserves of energy,

when sleep is needed, one of three things will happen:

1. We won't get to sleep at all.

2. We will go to sleep but then wake up in the early hours when the energy has been used up.

3. We will sleep all night but it will be a very restless sleep, one with a lot of dreams and turning over. This is usually more common with younger, fitter people.

The brain never really switches off when the reserves of energy are too low. It can't. It has to keep going, even though at a lower rate, to ensure that the vital energy is kept flowing to the organs that most require it. If the brain didn't keep going then all sorts of problems would follow.

One of the strange things about insomnia is that although sufferers very often can't sleep at night they have no trouble sleeping during the day (cat-napping), especially when they have other people around them. This is because one person's electrical field can influence another's. In other words the surplus energy of one is absorbed to affect the energy field of another. If the brain is starved of sleep and that person comes close to someone with a surplus of energy during the daytime, he will absorb from the other what he requires for the body to manage while his brain switches off in sleep to revitalise itself. This is something we have all experienced, especially under stress.

WEARINESS

As I explained earlier, an electrical current creates an electro-magnetic field and electromagnetic fields overcome gravitational pull. The more energy you have, the more easily you walk across the planet. The less energy you have the more difficult it is to get up and keep moving.

All life, animal and vegetable, has an electromagnetic field. If it didn't it wouldn't be able to pull away from the earth's gravitational pull. Every seed has its own electromagnetic (life) field. It is this energy field which allows the germinating plant to move up towards the sun and away from gravitational pull. The plants in your home are growing 'up' because of their life-field. If this field is weakened for any reason the plant begins to droop. Its ability to overcome gravity gradually weakens until finally, when its life-field is totally used up, it dies and falls back to earth.

As a seed's electromagnetic field drops, so does its vigour. We are the same. Our energy is our shield against gravitational forces and when that energy is insufficient we find getting out of chairs, walking and even standing are far more difficult. The more energy we have, the more easily we move about; the less energy we have the more difficult it becomes to move around. Furthermore, as the energy drops so the weight carried by our skeletal frame increases. This in turn causes us pain, especially in the legs and lower back, as downward pressure puts strain on the joints. A 15 stone man who is full of energy will be much lighter on his feet than a 10 stone man who is under stress.

MEMORY

Besides generating the body's energy, the brain also controls our mental functions. The brain is the body's computer and, like all computers needs a supply of electricity in order to function. To be fully functional, it requires energy to flow through it at exactly the right rate. Too little and it won't fully switch on; too much and it will switch off.

One of the common problems caused by stress is amnesia. Not serious memory loss, but just sufficient to cause embarrassment. When energy is low it becomes difficult to remember details, such as names and dates. Often it's put down to 'old age'. In most people it's nothing of the sort. It's just that, without sufficient electrical supply, the computer is failing to switch on. Furthermore it's just as difficult to get the computer to accept new information as it is to get stored information out. How often, when you feel tired, do you have difficulty concentrating? How often do you begin to read a book only to find that you can't recall the names of important characters before reaching the second page?

When you can't put information into your computer, and you can't retrieve information from it, you don't have enough detail on which to base decisions and so decision-making becomes very difficult. At this point we become impatient, bad-tempered or depressed to avoid being questioned. We lack the energy to respond quickly or efficiently.

ENERGY SOURCE

There is one question I always ask if a client comes to me, with some or all of the symptoms of stress. 'Do you take sugar?' They often answer 'No, I don't take it at all.' Experience has shown me that when people are on sugar-free diets, particularly in situations of stress, and they complain of feeling tired or drained they will have most of the symptoms listed above. Others with these symptoms are people in jobs or situations requiring a high level of concentration, responsibility or activity, such as lorry drivers, businessmen or athletes. These people are all exhibiting symptoms of low energy. I suppose the most extreme and sudden energy loss is caused by shock. A sudden release of energy is sometimes necessary to escape from a life-threatening situation. All of one's energies may be released in order to survive a period of extreme stress, such as the death of a loved one. How often it seems that the bereaved manage to cope until the anxiety that the death caused has ceased. Then they suddenly 'go to pieces'. Shock may also be caused by uncon-scious fear or trauma, such as an earlier operation which does not appear to have caused any physical problem.

Whatever the reason, if you have ever experienced shock you will know what a truly awful feeling it is. First sweating, then feeling terribly cold, stomach screwing up, etc. All these are extreme versions of the symptoms of stress. What are we told to do with someone in shock? Keep them warm and give them a cup of sweet tea. Why? Because the sugar in the tea brings them out of shock. It's the lack of energy to meet excessive demands which causes them to feel cold, muscles to tense up, the brain to go numb.

At this point every dietician worth his or her salt will be jumping up and down, raging about how bad sugar is for your health. According to Professor Eric Jequiers, who headed a team of Swiss scientists researching the effects of sugar on body weight at Lausanne University, the body uses up carbohydrates, sugar and starch within twenty-four hours and only 1 per cent turns to fat. However, if you are going to cut sugar out of people's diets you need to replace it with another energy source. So let's begin at the beginning.

Energy comes from the sun. If you doubt it, ask yourself how you feel when the sun is shining. Even those who suffer from stiff limbs or tiredness all seem to come alive on a sunny day. The sun's energy is electricity, and we all absorb it and utilise it. Fortunately for us, so do plants. Plants convert the sun's energy, through photosynthesis, into sugar. We eat the plants, and convert the sugar into glucose and glucose back into energy. I know it's a lot more complex than that but I think you get the picture. Without energy we die, or at best slow down. So why is sugar bad for us?

Professor Jequiers's investigations have shown that it is the ingredients sugar is mixed with which cause the problems. Chocolates, cakes and other sweetened foods usually contain large amounts of fat and it is the fat which causes the weight and health problems. Even so, I would still avoid sugar because of its complex molecular structure which makes it difficult for the body's digestive system to break it down. Only a small proportion of sugar in this form is readily converted to glucose. The rest, if the body has no need for it, does all the horrible things dieticians tell us it does, including being laid down as weight for another day. Whereas glucose, because of its very simple molecular structure, is easily and quickly assimilated into the body and utilised before any other available energy.

Hundreds of years ago before bank overdrafts, fast cars, time and motion studies, mortgages and the like we got all the energy we needed from the food we ate. But times have changed. Society is generally more competitive and more materialistic. We have created for ourselves an artificial environment that produces excessive levels of stress which require artificially high levels of energy In this situation we need to supplement our natural diet with increased levels of energy to meet the extra demands we make on ourselves. When our energy levels are not sufficient to meet those needs we are offered various artificial stimulants to make up the shortfall.

We take tranquillisers in order to slow ourselves down and reduce our need for energy, or sleeping tablets to chemically induce sleep, or stimulants to increase our energy to help us meet the demands of the twentieth century. Many turn to alcohol which is also a concentrated form of energy. After all, have you ever seen someone who is drunk having difficulty with sleep or feeling cold? Have you ever noticed how they don't hurt themselves when they fall? This is because gravitational pull is having less effect. Have you noticed how loose-limbed they are?

However, like other drugs, any advantage that may be gained in the beginning by drinking alcohol to, say, get to sleep or feel good, will quickly be lost, as the body begins to rely on alcohol to the exclusion of other forms of energy. At this point addiction takes over and the old problems return. The advantages are lost and one now has the added problem of alcohol or drug addiction.

WEIGHT

When someone comes to me with the symptoms of stress I always recommend large intakes of glucose over a short period. I have had doctors tell me it's a waste of time, but they use it themselves on patients who are seriously ill or recovering from the shock of an operation. (In fairness I know some doctors who do stock glucose.)

I usually experience some resistance from my female clients to the suggestion that they should take glucose for a week or so. They are usually overly concerned about their weight. As I point out, glucose is not habit-forming, it's not poisonous, and it's not fattening, as long as you need it. So just watch your weight and if you begin to put on a pound or so stop taking it. But nine out of ten don't put weight on, even at the 4-5 dessertspoons a day level which I recommend.

I remember one particular client who came to see me. She was over 16 stone and gaining (her expression not mine). I suggested she take up to 7 dessertspoons a day for a week and then come and see me again. She declared that she would sue me if she put on an ounce, especially as she had come about her weight in the first place. At the end of the week she returned, with a big smile and 7 pounds lighter. She continued to lose weight for several weeks, and as her weight loss began to slow up so she reduced her glucose intake.

The reason for this success was quite simple. The woman in question had all sorts of family problems and had been 'comfort eating'. She had acquired a sweet tooth because her body knew better than she did what it needed. Because of all her worries she was utilising energy faster than she was taking it in. She therefore began to eat cakes, chocolate, biscuits, anything with sugar in it to try and make up for the energy she was losing. Most of the sugar in these foods can't be converted into glucose fast enough to satisfy energy needs, so it is set aside for another day. But as her demand for energy was continuous, so she kept eating and her bodily reserves increased.

Once I put her on to glucose, which she instantly converted to energy, her need for sugar dropped and so did her comfort eating. She also began to utilise some of her sugar reserves.

Another factor also came into play here. As I said earlier, pulsed energy helps keep the muscles relaxed, taking pressure off the heart as well as helping it pump blood around the body. But the pumping action of the muscles also helps fluids flow back to the kidneys. Glucose can have a diuretic effect. In young people with very firm muscles too much glucose can cause constipation but in older people with softer muscle fibres it doesn't seem to do this. Their softer muscle tissue absorbs fluids when the pumping action of the muscles is insufficient to help move the fluids back towards the kidneys I would not recommend glucose as a diuretic, but where there is an obvious need for a high energy intake a diuretic effect will sometimes be noticed. If you believe you need a diuretic or any other form of health care you should always consult your doctor first. But ask yourself, have you cut sugar totally from your diet? And if so, where is your energy coming from?

So how much glucose would I recommend to treat stress? As a rule, 4-5 dessertspoons a day for a week or so. But it depends on the situation and the reason for the energy loss. If the only problem is insomnia I would suggest taking 1 heaped dessertspoon in water before going to bed. It will often work as well as any sleeping tablet. If the person concerned is waking in the night I suggest, again, the dessertspoonful in water, to be prepared and left by the bed, so if they do wake in the night all they have to do is drink the glucose and in about three to five minutes slide back into sleep.

For most people, I suggest they keep taking the 4-5 dessertspoons a day (that is, 1 when you get up, 1 mid-morning, 1 mid-afternoon and another in the evening) for about five to ten days. Naturally it goes without saying that none of these suggestions should be considered until you have discussed the problem with your doctor and he has more or less given up on you, and certainly not if you have any reason to believe that you might be diabetic. A diet that totally excludes any form of sugar is eventually going to lead to problems. I know because I see the results in my treatment room every day. Here is just one example:

Very recently I had a young man come to me with stomach cramps. He was a long-distance lorry driver and a few years earlier he had had an ileostomy (an operation to remove the large intestine) to try and overcome the continual stomach pains he was having. The pains continued after his operation and they opened him up a second time but could find nothing wrong. This time the doctors came to the conclusion that the pains were due to lesions around the earlier operation. Whatever the reason the stomach cramps continued and he was having to take time off from work. This put added pressure on him, as he was likely to lose his job and in the current economic climate it would be very difficult to find another job.

As he sat in the treatment room relating his story, it became more and more obvious that his only problem was stress, made worse by the fact that he was sitting bent forward for long periods every day, and I suspect eating his lunch as he drove along. The remedy was simple. I put him on to glucose. He came a second time a week later and all his pains had gone. For the first time in years he was sleeping soundly all night and the irritability and quick temper he had become prone to had completely gone. He was now beginning to enjoy life again. A very large percentage of the people who come to me need no more help than the occasional dessertspoonful of glucose.

Recommending glucose may not be what you expect of a healer, but why come to me for more energy when you can deal with the problem yourself? As a healer, I give the patient the means by which they heal themselves. It is a fallacy to believe that one person heals another. I don't wish anyone to become dependent upon me and the sooner they begin to heal without my help, the better.

INFERTILITY

Many, many illnesses are directly related to the electromagnetic field — that is the energy flow of the body. When this is weakened through shock, damage, fear or worry, illness occurs. It shows in symptoms as varied as cramp and cancer, backache and infertility.

I have often been asked to help with female infertility

problems. Each one of the women concerned had gone to their doctor first, and then through the usual routine of discussions with consultants and visits to the clinics. I treat these as straightforward healing situations but I always ask about tired muscles and cramp, feeling cold, difficulty sleeping etc. — in fact all the questions associated with stress — and nearly every time when I get around to the question about diet and sugar I get the same answer. Yes, they are on a diet. Or no, they don't take sugar. I always give the same reply .... 'I expect that's your problem, not enough energy.' The explanation I give goes something like this.

I used to manage farms and dairy units and in the winter when we needed to put the bull to the cows there would, in some years, be a problem because the cows wouldn't show sufficient interest. This made it difficult for the herdsman to recognise which cows needed to be separated from the herd for insemination. Even when the cows were inseminated it was very probable that they wouldn't conceive and the whole perform-ance would have to be repeated again. To a dairy farmer this was very costly, as he needs to produce a calf from each cow as near to every twelve months as possible.

The years in which this problem was most likely to occur were those following a poor summer, when the sunlight hours had been well below average. A cow's main diet is grass in one form or another, and during the winter months she will be feasting on grass harvested during the previous May and June. If during the growing time of April and May the number of sunny days had been below average, the growing grass wouldn't have had the opportunity to convert the sun's rays through photosynthesis, into sugar. Consequently sugar levels in the harvested grass would be low — very often several per cent lower than normal. When it became evident that this was going to be a problem we would buy-in drums of molasses and pour it along the feed troughs. It had a remarkable effect on the cows and conception rates could be guaranteed to improve almost immediately.

My advice to women with infertility is nearly always the same. Forget the diet (you are going to lose your figure anyway) and start taking glucose. It hardly ever fails. Healing also helps correct low energy levels, but it's a lot easier if the ladies correct their energy levels for themselves. This advice also applies in some instances to women who find they continually miscarry.

I have had women who have visited each week right through pregnancy because of a history of miscarrying. The healing was very effective but also time consuming, and when they have to travel sometimes over 100 miles in both directions it's not very practical. Now I just advise them to go on to glucose and let their doctor know what they are doing. The body is wonderfully self-regulating and if it decides that there isn't enough energy within its system to support a foetus then it will either refuse to conceive, or it will miscarry. A foetus is a collection of very rapidly dividing cells demanding nutritional priority before any of the mother's other bodily needs can be satisfied. If the energy is not there, then the body just sheds the hungry cells before they become too demanding.

Of course there are other reasons for infertility but I think this one is probably one of the main reasons and it's certainly worth considering first. Healing can get you into trouble though. One young woman rang and spoke to my wife to make an appointment. She said she had heard that I was good at helping ladies become pregnant. Would I help her? As an afterthought she asked, 'Can my husband come as well? I want him to see how it's done.' All in a day's work.

— 4 —

Flight Path

Apart from times of stress, there are periods in our lives when our energy may be insufficient to meet our daily needs. Each and every one of us is going to fall into first one and then another of these categories. The first category is infancy, the second is adolescence and the third old age, three stages in our 'flight path' through life. You can define old age as you wish. I know of some people who are old at fifty and some who are young at ninety.

CHILDHOOD

When we are very young — in fact up to our teens — our brains are undeveloped and not capable of generating sufficient energy for our own needs. The energy required by the multiplying cells is extraordinary and there is no way an infant can get all the energy it needs from its own resources. It therefore depends heavily on its parents, usually its mother, to supply those needs.

Anyone who has ever brought up a family of young children will tell you how tiring they are. Young children make incredible demands on adults around them. The younger they are, the greater their cell multiplication rate and the greater their need for energy. In the first section I explained how electricity was a necessary stimulant to cell division, and division or multiplication of cells is especially necessary in a fast-growing child. In fact their whole system, mental and physical is working at a faster speed than that of an adult. Add to that the fact that their food is not always of the right high-energy type, and you will see that a youngster's demand for life-giving energy often has to be met from an external source.

The extra energy a child needs comes in the form of radiated energy which is picked up from its parents' electromagnetic field. In order to absorb this energy the child needs to bond quickly with the adult upon whom it is going to rely for that extra supply. Bonding means coming into harmony with, and by being in harmony with an adult the youngster will automatically be able to absorb and utilise the surplus energy from its parent's radiating energy field. A child doesn't only need milk and security from its parents. Its first instinctive tie to adults is not one of love but one of selfish need for the energy of life which will cause it to grow and develop faster than it would if left to itself.

Any stock farmer will tell you that a calf which is left with its dam for a month or so will, during that time, become a far bigger and stronger animal than one taken from the cow at birth and reared on the bucket. And this is the case even if every other part of the rearing is identical. It's nothing to do with the amount of milk either calf may receive; it's to do with that extra x factor which we call by various names such as love, caring and tenderness.

It all adds up to the same thing — close contact between mother and child, allowing a transfer of energy from one to the other. This is what bonding is all about. With our modern tendency towards bottle feeding and the busy life many parents have to lead away from the home, many children are denied a close bonded relationship in the very early stages of life. Lack of bonding prevents children experiencing harmony with the thoughts of their parents and this becomes very apparent later in their lives.

Of course children don't absorb energy exclusively from their parents; they will take it from anyone who is prepared to give it to them. As an example, let's say you decide to have a party. So as not to disturb the baby you put him in the furthest and quietest part of the house. But within an hour or so he will be crying, trying to attract attention. His energy will have been depleted and he will be unable to sleep. Now put the baby in the room where the party is in full swing, where there is lots of noise and activity, and within minutes he will be fast asleep. And what's more he is likely to sleep right through the night. This is because in a party atmosphere there is an abundance of surplus energy about. People are happy, excited, positive and the baby soaks it up.

I just cannot over-emphasise the importance of continued close contact for babies. The sooner they bond and harmonise with their parents' energy, particularly their mothers', the sooner they will relax and become part of the family group. This is just another form of healing. Babies put into crêches or left with friends while mother is at work all day are not going to harmonise easily or bond with their parents and so sometimes will not as readily grow as one of the family. They may grow up to be outside the family group, possibly even disruptive and aggressive, or sullen and withdrawn. This is because the energy the baby should be getting from the parents is not forthcoming and so, if it is to survive, the isolated child needs to become independent quickly or get its energy from someone else. Managing without its parents' energy at such an early age causes the child to become out of harmony with its parents. The child then remains alone and independent because it hasn't learned how to function as part of a harmonious group.

Cot Death

I believe there is a link between a child's energy level and its ability to survive. Physically a baby can be perfect but if for some reason or other its energy level falls below that required to hold it into its body it will begin to have an 'out-of-the-body' experience. If the energy level is not quickly recharged then the spirit or soul of the baby will not be able to re-enter its body which will cease to function. This has nothing to do with how the child is loved. It is a form of disability.

Babies just don't have the capacity to generate sufficient energy of their own which is why they seldom sleep right through the night. They wake and cry to attract attention and a cuddle in order to replace their lost energy. Without energy we can't sleep, because the brain needs to keep working to generate energy. If we do go on sleeping when our energy is completely depleted we move out of our bodies and may die. I remember very clearly when I was a baby how I used to play games by leaving my body, but after a while I struggled to resist the experience.

Parent/Child Relationships

All babies need the close association of a caring adult. Not any adult, but one from whom they can feel love and with whom they can bond. Many adults suffer neurosis as a direct result of being denied a childhood bonding relationship with a parent.

Only recently I have helped two women who had suffered all their lives — one is now in her fifties and the other in her late thirties — because when they were born they were cared for by people other than their mothers. In one case it was the grandmother and in the other case it was the father. Because the father was out of work and the wife was working it was sensible for him to stay at home and care for their baby. However both women grew up to be neurotic and during healing sessions they said they felt that they weren't wanted by their mothers.

For nine months the unborn child had been growing inside a body which was responsible for the electricity of the growing child's life-force. The mother had also become responsible for the frequency of the electromagnetic force. Suddenly, at birth, the child is separated from that electromagnetic energy. But it needs to be kept in close contact with it for several months while it creates and forms its own independent thinking processes.

Imagine, if you can, how you would feel if the person emotionally closest to you, the one with whom you share your love, were to leave you or die, and within minutes be replaced by a total stranger who came into your life and tried to take the place of the one you have lost. At best you would feel a need to keep a distance. It takes time to build up a close relationship. I also suggest that if the one with whom you are sharing a deep emotional love was suddenly to say to you, 'From now on I have chosen someone else to love you in my place,' you would feel horrified and rejected. This is exactly what happens to babies who are taken over to be cared for by someone other than their mother soon after they are born. Today's children are generally very independent and therefore selfish, they need to be to survive, but they will have problems in later life, because they won't have learnt how to work with others or help others. If they don't learn how to share the energy of a group they won't learn how to give. Bonding means learning to give as well as take. I realise that not all mothers are lucky enough to be able to spend all the time they would like with their babies, but provided they are able to nurse their babies for the first few months all will be well. It is in the first few months, particularly immediately after birth, that close association with mother is so essential.

It is the feeling of rejection which babies feel as well as the loss of mother's energy which can cause insecurity in later life. For children who are adopted and who grow up in close, loving relationships with their adopted parents the initial feelings of rejection are usually soon forgotten. What is essential is for the mother or father to explain to the baby why they need to be away and when they will be coming back.

I recall a man who at birth was separated from his mother for several days because of her need for medical attention. He told me that all his life he had had a dread of being separated from his family. He was constantly running away from school to be at home. When he married he continued to live close to his mother and when she died his grief was extreme. He recalled during a healing session the fear and rejection he had felt at birth when he had been separated from his mother and no one had explained to him the reasons why. This baby whose life was measured in hours rather than days was already making logical judgements. If you need to be separated from your baby explain why. It will do much to ease their insecurity.

Our thoughts are generated through the brain to become, as surplus, an electromagnetic field. Because energy is the product of the brain, it has the thought imprints of the parent or parents in it. Therefore the child receiving this energy will develop a pattern of thinking very much akin to those who are supplying the energy.

'Give me the child until he is seven and I will show you the man.' So goes the Jesuit saying, and it's quite easy to see the truth of this. The child develops according to the thoughts in the energy it is fed on.

Hyperactive Children

I've treated hyperactive children who haven't been able to rest, who have needed to be on the go all the time, and they nearly always fall asleep in my arms. I'm sure that for some of these children the problem is that they haven't bonded with their parents and so are unable to absorb the surplus energy the parents radiate. Their brains then have to work at full stretch to ensure that they generate and create as much energy as they can. Although their symptoms show an excess of energy I'm sure if we could measure bioelectrical fields we would find that some of these children are low on energy, not high, which is why they readily sleep when I hold them. Crying, restless children have always quietened down in my presence; even teething pains seem to lose their sting when I'm about. I believe this is because I give their system a boost of bioelectrical energy which takes away the need to cry or attract attention. Of course not all problems with children are caused by insufficient energy but they do respond well to healing. Perhaps this is why in our sunless country growing children with high energy levels crave sweets or sugar in other forms.

Heart Problems

Babies are the easiest of all ages to treat. They are totally trusting, totally dependent upon energy transference, and their whole life support system is fully charged with an ambition to live. One of the youngest children I have ever treated was just seven weeks old. The poor little mite had a heart and lung defect. For some reason his blood was not getting to his lungs in large enough quantities and, as the weeks went by and his need for oxygen increased, so his strength and life-force became weaker.

When he first came to me he had hardly grown, he was weak and a horrible colour. I held him in my hands for about twenty minutes once a week for four weeks. By the eleventh week of his life he had totally changed. Originally he had been given a life expectancy of about thirteen weeks. After the first four visits I didn't need to see him again but I did meet his grandmother about eighteen months later at a lecture I was giving. She came to see me at the end of the evening to tell me that her grandson was growing into a strong healthy boy.

ADOLESCENCE

Students often live in a state of sustained stress, especially those who are living away from home for the first time in their lives. They are keenly aware that much is expected of them. Such is the pressure from friends and family that they are often in a state of anxiety even before they leave. Unfortunately many young people leaving home to begin college or university education have been ill-prepared for the task. It is unlikely they will have been given any advice on independence or how to maintain it. Until they leave home, usually in their late teens, these young adults have been receiving regular supplies of energy from the home environment. Few demands were made of them and they were easily able to maintain a strong bioelectrical field. Then they suddenly find themselves away from the protective, harmonious atmosphere of home, and its strength and energy. Worse, they are now in a hostile environment. There is no protective energy here; they are now totally alone, and responsible for attracting or creating energy for themselves. Stress makes greater demands on them than ever before and so their utilisation of energy is vastly increased.

As if that did not pose enough difficulties, they are grouped with others who are also trying to adjust to a new situation. In doing so they will be attracted to others who have similar thought frequencies. This causes the positive, strong and independent ones to group together and the negative, weak and dependent to form other groupings. The strong and independently minded students go on to boost each other but what of the negative or weaker students? This group requires far more energy than it can supply. If they do not quickly learn how to become positive and independent, the other, stronger students will shun them.

This is a very basic instinct. It can be seen in every playground, at every age. In the wild, animals who live in communities share the energy they have, the one with the most energy usually becoming leader of the pack. This is natural enough, as this is the one the others feel drawn to. It's what we call charisma — surplus energy.

If one of the pack becomes ill or weak it begins to make demands on the whole group and if it is allowed to remain within the group then the whole unit will eventually begin to weaken and be put at risk. So if, through age or illness, the energy level of an individual in the team drops to a level where it begins to affect the others they will hound it out of the group, and force it away to fend for itself or die.

Bullying in a playground is very similar. It is always the weaker ones who are picked on. Those with the most energy are usually the most popular because they draw the others to themselves. The problem with a playground situation is that the weaker ones can only be forced away as far as the fence and in intensive grouping situations this is still within the sensitive range of other children. I've seen sick cows in herds of cattle treated terribly by the others because they are unable to get away due to the boundary fence. The only way to save them is to bring them into a pen, away from the herd until they recover their full strength.

To strengthen such children, send them to a healer to boost their energy and confidence. Healing truly has an amazing effect on children lacking confidence. After a few sessions from a healer with counselling skills a shy, bullied child will grow confident and assertive and, more important, be accepted by its peers.

Depression

Over the months the weaker student becomes more and more negative, and studies become a nightmare because his brain lacks the energy to comprehend, retain or recall information. Without these facilities at his disposal, decision-making becomes almost impossible. At this point depression begins to take over, depression being an energy level so low that the effort needed to rise up again is too great without help. The student might now turn to drugs or alcohol which will give a short-term boost to his energy but which are unfortunately also addictive. In this situation the student may become deeply depressive, even suicidal.

I realise that this is an extreme example, but far too many students are near this danger line at some stage of their college life. And it's not only students who go through this hell. Doctors' surgeries are full of people whose energy levels have sunk well below a safe level. A lot of people in need of medical help wouldn't have reached that point if they had been able to recognise the symptoms of stress at an earlier stage, before it produced physical symptoms. If they had been able to see what was happening and had visited a good healer for a few sessions, just to boost their batteries, they might have remained fit and well. They would almost certainly benefit from taking glucose.

OLD AGE

The other obvious period when our energy is likely to be below what we require for an active life is in our later years. We know that as the brain ages it loses cells which are not replaced. Our generator therefore becomes less efficient, no matter how fit, positive and healthy we may be. The older we become, the more we notice the symptoms of stress creeping up on us. We have difficulty getting off to sleep or we only sleep for short periods and cat-nap during the day when other people are about. Our muscles stiffen and our joints tighten, making standing up straight and walking difficult. In fact any form of exercise becomes increasingly difficult as we get older. And we feel the cold more, as energy levels drop.

Circumstances experienced during our lives create the conditions from which we emerge old or young. A group of elderly people living together will tend to have their individual energies reduced to an equal level. Someone with more than usual energy and vitality who goes into a home for the elderly will soon be reduced to the same energy level as the others. This is because the other residents will all be trying to boost their own energy unknowingly and unwittingly, by drawing on those who have more, thus reducing everybody's energy to a common level. I think people who work with, and care for the elderly, especially in nursing homes, should have their hours limited by law for their own protection. They should also be paid much higher wages for doing such wonderful work (work which the rest of us don't want to do, or the old people's homes would not be so full). I believe they would be able to do their work in a far happier frame of mind, benefiting everyone, if these conditions were imposed. We would all gain because one day many of us are going to need the services of a nursing home ourselves.

RELATIONSHIPS

As I've explained elsewhere, our bioelectricity, energy, is transferable between people and it's this which begins the process of lifting someone free of depression, even if there is an emotional or spiritual background to the problem. We can't overcome any emotional or spiritual problem unless our energy levels are adequate to deal with the associated stress.

Let's take the situation of a young daughter who is caring for an elderly parent or parents, especially if the parents are negative in their attitudes. Negative attitudes cause endless difficulties both for those who harbour them and those who need to care for the ones with the negative attitudes. Negative people absorb energy from others. They are quite incapable of creating enough for themselves, so they literally draw it in from others around them. If you have ever been near anyone who is doing this you will know what I mean.

I have seen cases where the elderly parent has taken practically all the life and spirit from the younger relative caring for them. I remember one case in particular where a dutiful daughter started to call in on her mother for company and do what she could to help, as the father had recently died. But the mother was expecting energy in equal amounts to that which her husband had provided and she began to make more demands upon her daughter until the girl was spending all her spare time at her mother's house. The daughter became more and more drained and tired. Even this wasn't enough for the mother who now wanted the exhausted daughter to move in with her.

Because the daughter had very little energy left she hadn't the emotional strength to put up any resistance to the idea. The daughter had now become a virtual slave, without either the mother or herself realising it. The mother's health remained strong and she couldn't understand why her daughter was always so tired. By the time the mother died, many years later, the daughter had herself become an old woman, although still young in years. Her energy had been drained from her for so long that she had gone past the point of recovery. I see this so often, the energy of one supplementing the energy of another to the point where dependence becomes total and the giving becomes life threatening.

In a normal marriage situation both partners become dependent upon each other for energy, meaning that their electromagnetic fields combine so there is an interchange of energy, a dependence which goes beyond a practical need and reaches deep into the emotional levels. This is a wonderful and much desired situation in any marriage, but when partners become so close that they lose their independence then the grief and loss they experience when one or the other dies is excessive. It can compare to the withdrawal symptoms suffered by someone trying to give up drugs. Grief is always worse in cases of total emotional dependency and not much better in shared dependency.

The problem begins the moment one of the partners leaves or dies, so reducing the overall bioelectrical field by half at least. Even a dying person is producing and radiating a field even though it may only be a weak one, and we never realise how much part of the other we have become until they are no longer there. The loss of this energy makes the grief so much worse, and it can turn into depression which unfortunately often continues for a long time. When someone's level of energy is so low, it really is difficult for them to recharge their batteries on their own. The situation is just like that of a new car with a flat battery: mechanically perfect, but it can't bring itself to life until connected to another battery which will get it going again.

Healing is truly wonderful in these situations and a half hour session can work miracles. All that is necessary is for the healer to impart healing love which revitalises every one of the millions of cells which go to make up the body. People who have spent a whole lifetime on their own don't usually have the same sort of problems adjusting to changed situations. Companionship of any sort provides a lot more than shared interest; it provides life in the form of shared energy fields.

I also believe that when a loved one is lost so is the benefit of human touch. To be touched or held by another is a wonderful and necessary thing because it releases the pent-up emotions of grief, stress or depression. At the same time it allows the person to receive energy as love in the place of these negative emotions, but it often needs a direct touching contact to achieve this. One of the problems with our society is that we are often embarrassed to put our arms around a despondent, lonely or grieving friend. This is a very sad fact, and one of the things most missed by the grieving or lonely is to be touched, kindly and lovingly, by another human being. Such a simple thing to do.

Sometimes depression is caused by moving away from friends, a familiar workplace or some other situation where people were utilising energy other than their own. Take a man of sixty-five. Until the day he retires he is fully employed and working with a group of colleagues. The mental activity involved in thinking generates a fair amount of bioelectricity but because of his age he is most likely existing on the electromagnetic field produced by his working colleagues. Once retired and away from his friends and the activity of the workplace he is effectively cut off from his supply of energy. He is no longer able to recharge himself from the surplus his friends were radiating.

His wife, on the other hand, who was probably used to being on her own and independent, is unaffected by the change except probably to notice that her husband is now becoming a drain on her emotions. How long she will tolerate this situation or change to accommodate him depends very much on the relationship. If it is close they will both adjust. If they are not so close and he has not built up any leisure activities he's likely to just sit around and fade away. This may not be depression in the true sense, but it is one facet of it.

People who have worked as part of a team or in a factory or office all their lives are more dependent on other people and a community lifestyle than country people who rely more on nature and not necessarily other people for their life-force. Nature is alive with energy. Every plant, every tree has its own bioelectrical field and those of us who have spent most of our lives as one with this wonderful life-force seldom suffer the stresses created by living in a town. The bioelectrical field is the x-factor which makes life worthwhile, even possible. And the stronger it is the greater our ability to think and act as an independent person. But as our energy decreases we become less and less able to control our thoughts and actions.

When retirement is approaching, it really isn't very sensible to move away from the neighbourhood you have settled into. You will have become dependent on the energy of that area and bonded with it. To move into a new environment will cause problems in adjusting to new bioelectrical fields with which you may not be able to harmonise. In addition the type of energy available might be totally unsuitable to the demands you make of it. People who are in harmony with the life-forces of a city are not usually able to adjust to harmonising with totally different life-forces in the country, especially if they wait until retirement to make the change. For these reasons, people often weaken and die within months when they move to new districts late in life.

Loneliness is a type of depression, a longing to share life with someone who can contribute to your need for energy. Such

71

situations can be affected positively by healing but unfortunately this often leads to dependency upon the healer. Healing is supposed to create independence, not create dependence. But it is excellent as a short term boost to lift someone so that they can make a fresh start. As I have said, physical depression is an almost total lack of energy, sometimes brought about by shock (which drains the system too quickly) or by an energy-sapping illness. People suffering from these problems need personal attention from positive friends to help them restore their own energy levels so they can become independent again. We are all healers at some time in our lives especially when we give our time and attention to others.

PART II

THE AUTO PILOT

Healing the Mind and Emotions

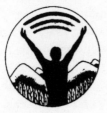

Emotion is the product of the subconscious computer, which is always active even during sleep and when necessary it takes over from logical thinking to protect the body from what it believes to be impending danger.

The computer has three main functions. Maintenance and repair, producing programs for daily living which we call habits, and protecting us from danger.

Maintenance and repair begins the moment the foetus becomes independent of its mother's computer. Habits are learned from casual activities which when repeated become programs which we use without having to relearn, such as riding a bike. Protection is learnt from situations of extreme emotion such as fear or shock. In this section we shall see how to understand the coded messages our computer uses to protect us from what it considers to be impending danger. Unless we can interpret the messages our computer displays as symptoms, we are likely to treat as illness a subconscious message of warning.

— 5 —

The Computer

More and more people are moving away from orthodox medicine and towards the new alternative or complementary therapies now available. I think one of the reasons for this is that doctors find it easier to treat the symptoms of a patient's illness than spend time searching for the cause. And in the majority of cases you will not find the cause in physical symptoms.

THE SUBCONSCIOUS

Most health problems have a subconscious origin. In other words at a subconscious level we bring psychosomatic illness upon ourselves to attract attention, or to overcome or avoid some kind of emotional trauma. Not deliberately, of course. In fact the sufferer will never be aware that they are the direct cause of their own sufferings.

I use the term 'psychosomatic' rather than 'psychological' because people think the term 'psychological' means they are making it up or deliberately causing themselves injury which is of course nonsense. At a conscious level people suffering from psychosomatic disorders are no more aware of what's causing their problem than anyone else. The pain or discomfort they experience is very real, but it is most unlikely that a doctor will be able to diagnose a psychosomatic problem unless he has in-depth knowledge of the family and more than the usual five minutes to listen to all his patient's problems. Even then, a lot of intuition is called for. One thing is absolutely certain. No tablets or drugs, etc. are likely to produce a cure, and if they do then the subconscious will probably either overcome the cure or create another illness. In these situations treating symptoms is a waste of time. It's the cause that needs to be treated, which is why drug therapy is so ineffectual.

If the subconscious has reason to believe that the body is in some way threatened then it will set about producing symptoms of illness in order to bring its worries to the attention of logical consciousness. It does this so that those from whom it seeks help or security are made aware of its needs. And it achieves its aim by changing the body's chemicals, its electrical frequencies or its physiology to produce a symptom which will attract attention. There are those who will say it is ridiculous to suggest that the subconscious can cause a cell to become something different from that which its own DNA coding has instructed it to become. But this is exactly what the subconscious, or the spirit controlling it, can do. Note how someone's character can change their physical features.

If you doubt this ask yourself what happens at the site of an injury. Let's say a muscle is damaged in an accident, torn, mutilated and partially ripped away. Immediately the body gets to work to stem the flow of blood. Then it discards the dead or useless tissue. It goes on to produce a complete programme of selected cell engineering, including making muscle cells, vein or artery cells, skin cells and a whole host of other types, until the wound is completely healed. How does the body know what sort of cell is required at the injury site and in what order? How does it know how to boost its production of cells in the right sequence at just that one spot and turn some into specialised muscle cells, others into blood vessel cells?

If the subconscious can re-program a complete production

system for a specified time to create a particular effect in a local area, it shouldn't have much difficulty producing a basic non-specialised cell to create a different effect, one we call cancer. Nor will it have any difficulty producing multiple sclerosis or a whole host of other physical symptoms. It has the power to change the DNA coding of any cell should it consider it necessary for its purposes. The problem is that the subconscious decides for itself what is good or bad for the body it is responsible for, and very often it overrides the wishes of the spirit which is supposed to be controlling it.

Spiritual healing gets right to the spirit to give it the strength to combat the arrogant subconscious. The subconscious has total control over our health and emotions unless it is controlled. It alone decides what is good for us and what isn't. It alone decides when the body needs rest and when it doesn't. Push the body too hard and the subconscious will produce the symptoms of stress as an early warning. If you have a difficulty ahead which is causing you problems, believe me, the subconscious will try and find a way out of it for you. If you find yourself in a situation which at an earlier age caused trauma the subconscious will send you warnings to be careful. If the same situation arises again it will produce a set of symptoms such as phobia or panic.

Doctors with an arsenal of chemicals at their disposal find it relatively simple to prescribe a course of drugs which will subdue the symptoms. But suppressing symptoms does not cure the problem. As long as the cause remains, the subconscious will produce another set of symptoms.

It is just not good enough to say to a patient symptoms he is displaying are due to cancer, or multiple sclerosis or arthritis. To do so is nonsense. Symptoms are not caused by multiple sclerosis. Multiple sclerosis is just a fancy medical name for a set of symptoms. So all the doctor is doing when he tells you that your symptoms are due to this or that condition is identify the name of the symptoms. He has not found or identified the cause.

It's like saying that cancer is caused by a malignant cell. No it's not. Cancer is the name given to a malignant cell. But that is not the cause, it is a symptom. Ask your doctor what caused the cell to become malignant and he might say 'a chemical change in the body'. But that is not the cause either so ask again and he might say 'a shock' in which case we are perhaps getting closer, but we still haven't got to the cause. Doctors very, very rarely identify the cause; they just find more and more symptoms. Unless the cause of the symptoms can be identified, the symptoms will appear again, or in another form if they are treated with drug therapy to mask or suppress them. This is especially true when the cause is an emotional one.

Let's be really clear about this because it is essential to understand this point if healing is to be successful. It is not cancer which kills but the cause of the cancer. It is not arthritis which causes the painful swelling in joints. Arthritis is the name given to the symptoms of painful, swollen joints. To beat it, you need to know what caused the symptoms. If you really want to confuse your doctor, ask him what caused the swelling. Then ask him what caused that and then what caused that and so on. You will never get to the cause, just a succession of symptoms. To be fair to the doctor, he's unlikely to know enough about the life of his patient to even guess at the cause.

Lets look at an example. A young boy called Tom, aged fourteen, came with his mother to see if I could do anything about a condition he had which the doctors called Osteo Chondritis Dirsecans. This was a condition in which the blood, for some unknown reason, was not flowing as it should to the knees, with the result that the knee-caps were not growing. In fact they were beginning to flake and break up. This is how it was described to me by his mother. He had seen a consultant just a week or so earlier and been told that there was nothing that could be done, as it was a condition, not a disease, but that maybe when he had finished growing all might come right.

The condition was very painful and Tom wasn't able to straighten his legs properly. Obviously any form of sport was out of the question. I sat him down in front of me and held his ankles to harmonise with his energy. I do this to 'tune in' to people's subconscious thoughts. It took only a few minutes to realise why this condition had come about. Tom is one of those gifted youngsters who is a natural sportsman — excellent at swimming, football, athletics, gymnastics, golf and I suppose anything else he cares to try his hand at. He had decided at a very early age that sport would be his career. He planned to go on to college and qualify as a sports teacher. So I asked him what he wanted to do. That might sound like a silly question but it had the desired effect. He didn't answer. I asked him again. Still no answer. Then I asked him what he wanted to do *now* and straight away he said, 'Engineering.'

At this point I explained to Tom that inside each of us there is a master controller called our subconscious. This controller is totally and absolutely responsible for our health, both emotional and physical, but it will always put our contentment, or rather what it thinks is best for our contentment, first. This controller is responsible for seeing that our heart beats correctly, our lungs pump regularly, and that oxygen is carried around in the blood to where it's needed; it controls our circulation system, and the number of red and white cells that we have. It sends white cells to fight or defend those parts of the body under attack from disease. It is responsible for the repair and maintenance of every area of our body, from the rate at which our hair grows to extracting the nutrients from the foods we eat.

This same controller is responsible for the chemical balance in our body, for deciding what we see or don't see, even for which sounds we hear or don't hear. In fact if I were to list every individual responsibility of our subconscious controller I couldn't tell you in a non-stop twenty-four hour talk what our controller does each one-billionth of a second. This remarkable organiser of our lives is totally dedicated to our well being and contentment.

When Tom changed his mind, as youngsters do, and began

to feel that he no longer wanted to be a sportsman there shouldn't have been any difficulty. But if you are gifted and everyone is expecting great things of you, it is difficult to disappoint people, especially if you are sensitive and don't wish to hurt anyone. His parents had put a lot of time and energy into helping him to achieve what had been his ambition, with extra lessons, trips to athletic meetings, etc. His gym master at school had also given up his weekends and evenings to coach and train him. So many people had done so much to help Tom in his ambitions that when those ambitions changed he just didn't know how to tell them. It was then that his subconscious controller took over. Recognising Tom's dilemma, the controller decided to reduce the blood supply to the knees, knowing very well what the outcome would be. It wasn't very long before Tom was in acute pain and unable to take part in any sport.

After I had explained all this to Tom I took his ankles and held his legs straight out in front of him. His pain had practically gone and his legs were almost straight. His mother was astounded. In less than half an hour Tom was more or less back to normal. Of course it would take a little while for his knees to heal but otherwise his condition was cured. Why? Quite simply because Tom's controller knew that now his mother knew of his changed ambitions there would be no need to cause a malfunction in his knees. A visit to the consultant three weeks later confirmed that Tom's knees were healing fast and no treatment would be necessary.

Multiple Sclerosis

One of the infirmities I always have great sympathy for is multiple sclerosis (MS). In the past I treated many people with MS and wasted my time, and theirs, simply because I hadn't identified the deeper cause of their symptoms. I didn't cure a single case of MS, though I can claim to have helped many, until I began to enquire into the spirit of the patients.

In those people where the MS has not been long term, I have had some quite remarkable successes, especially where it is a case of the subconscious copying the symptoms of genuine MS. What I mean is that the subconscious seems to need a model on which to base its symptoms. If there had never been an original, disease-produced, MS then the subconscious would have had nothing to use as a model. The problem for both patients and doctors is knowing which is subconsciously produced and which is disease-produced, because physically there is no difference. The subconscious can produce an exact replica of the genuine problem.

I don't suppose anyone will ever know how many MS cases have evolved because of disease and how many because of trauma. But one thing is certain, the effects of a subconsciously produced problem, in this case MS, will eventually cause the same physical symptoms. Even the subconscious eventually loses control of the problem it has produced so that it can no longer be distinguished from the disease-produced version. If the condition is left for too long without attention any damage becomes permanent and the condition becomes irreversible.

The subconscious can and does cause irreparable injury to the body it is supposed to be looking after. And if it is to be persuaded to stop its damaging action then one has to enquire of the spirit why it is doing it. No, am not saying that MS sufferers are deliberately, consciously, causing their own suffering or pretending to have disabilities. The subconscious is taking action in the only way it knows, producing a reaction to satisfy or protect an emotional need. What action this keeper of our emotions takes is more or less beyond our control.

How do you tell someone who can't walk without support, and who was diagnosed as having MS ten years earlier, that they need not have any of these symptoms if they choose not to? It has to be done very carefully and I would never attempt it unless I knew my patient's thoughts and attitudes very thoroughly. Again, this is where being a healer helps.

I don't always see or hear the physical person in front of me, because sometimes I need to see the spirit or their emotional personality. I have come to the conclusion that for healing to be at its most effective it has to be accompanied by a great deal of empathy for the client and their emotional needs. I have had clients whose only barrier to recovery was the responsibility that would become theirs once fully fit. And I have given healing to clients whose illness, and in this I'm not just referring to MS, was mainly the result of not knowing how to challenge a parent or spouse.

Our subconscious is wonderfully inventive when faced with overwhelming odds of fear or competition. However, once the challenge is recognised and discussed, the debilitating symptoms will lift and the one affected will feel as if some great weight has been taken from their shoulders.

I have noticed that many of the MS cases I have been involved with have improved when problems concerning close relationships have been sorted out. I remember one lady who told me that after years of looking after her husband his MS suddenly cleared up when he met someone else, and another lady told me that her MS more or less cleared up when she decided not to be bullied by her husband. The point of all this is that in each of these cases the patient had been positively diagnosed as having MS and the only reason given for overcoming it was recognising that it was trauma-induced in the first place.

Of course, not all MS is psychosomatic and, anyway, much of that which is has gone on for too long and the damage caused to the nervous system has become permanent. But there must be a substantial number of cases, such as those I've outlined, which, if treated early enough, would respond to sympathetic healing.

I also know others who wouldn't be able to face the trauma which is the true cause of their illness and I don't have the authority, secular or spiritual, to make that decision for them. I remember one such patient. After two visits I told her I would cure her in six weeks. A look of delight crossed her face, and

I never saw her again. She gave all sorts of excuses but some people truly cannot manage without their problem. When we recognise this we have no right to take it from them without first dealing with whatever it is that causes such deep fear. And sometimes it is not necessarily in the best interests of the patient to have the cause of that fear brought to the surface.

Now I know that a lot of you will be thinking, this isn't healing, it's just good psychology. If you think that try telling someone in pain or with an infirmity that it's all in the subconscious and that their physical symptoms are mind-induced. If you manage to get away without a bloody nose you will have done well. To start with, it's doubtful if anyone who is in pain or ill is going to believe you. Even if they do grudgingly accept that you might be correct they are at best going to be irritated, especially as telling them achieves nothing.

What makes it possible for a healer to get away with it is that we commune with the patient's spirit as soon as they come through the door and this changes the whole situation. Many doctors have tried to tell patients that their problems are psychological, only to lose the patient's faith and trust. Healing isn't just a matter of putting 'healing hands' around someone; it's about giving them a glimpse of their own inner world.

One thing about healing is that the only tools I use are under the client's control and unless my clients trust me, and the help I give, I can't even begin to help them overcome their problems. I can't say it often enough. People heal themselves; doctors and healers are only there to help them succeed. Cases like these will not easily respond to drugs or surgery but if they do then the subconscious will just produce another set of new symptoms to express its repressed trauma.

The following is a letter I received from a lady who was able, with the help of healing, to release the emotions which were causing her cancer:

It was in June 1988 that I had part of my thyroid removed, and it was discovered that I had a very rare form of cancer. Everything had gone well until a week before Christmas 1991 when I discovered a lump in my neck. After courses of antibiotics and visits to the dentist to eliminate any infections, I was admitted to hospital in March 1992 for the removal of the lump.

Three weeks later I was back at the Outpatients Clinic, to be told by a doctor that the lump was a secondary from my thyroid cancer, but he did not know what to do as the consultant was on holiday, so I would have to make an appointment for a week's time. I hardly ate anything or slept during that time, but somehow managed to cope, and arrived back at the Outpatients Department a week later.

This time I saw the consultant, who told me he was sorry about the results, but he had only seen them that morning and did not know what to do. He thought he might send me to a London hospital, to see a specialist there who was an expert on the thyroid gland. But he was not sure whether he was in the country or not, so I was to go home and not worry and come back again in ten day's time.

It was then that I decided I needed help other than the medical profession.

On my first visit to Malcolm, he advised me to do as the specialist suggested and I would be all right, the cancer would go. But I had another problem that was causing me to be like I was, and would I like to talk about it. I had a problem. My husband had died eighteen months ago, and during that time I had put on a brave face, bottled everything up inside me and never grieved properly for him. What a relief it was to talk to someone, and get rid of all those pent-up feelings and emotions. I went back to see Malcolm again two days after my first visit, and I was a different person. I was happy, relaxed and I knew that I was going to be all right. On this visit Malcolm suggested that I had further investigations before I had any more treatment as the cancer had now gone.

Eventually I was admitted to a London hospital in July 1992, where various x-rays and scans were performed and all the results came back the same, no evidence of cancer detected.

J.S.

Emotional Problems

Healers treat many emotional problems, allowing the client to release stress and tension from the subconscious by relaxing the logical consciousness to the meditative state. When his electromagnetic field has been stilled by the healer the client will often involuntarily release pent-up emotions. Sometimes these emotions are lying just below the surface, only held in check by a resisting consciousness. But in the meditative state induced by healing, the barrier holding back the emotions is released and they come gushing out. It isn't always tears of unhappiness which are released. Sometimes it's rage and anger, and sometimes deep peace and contentment. The healer doesn't create the emotions; they are already there ready and waiting. I'm often told, 'You make me feel so happy,' But it's nothing to do with me. That contentment was already there, even if they hadn't realised it. An example illustrates this point.

A woman of about forty-five, divorced (let's call her Jane), came to see me with pains in her legs, back, arms and almost everywhere else. Not crippling pains, just general aches which seemed to move from one part of the body to another. She had had the usual tests and heard the well-worn phrase 'It's your age'. Anyway, Jane, who was certainly not the sort to feel sorry for herself, was becoming more and more distressed about her continual aches and pains.

I decided to start with her feet and legs. As soon as I put my hands around her ankles she began to shake and tremble from her toes, up through her legs on through her back and down her arms. I felt my own force-field beginning to totally overwhelm hers. I knew that I was putting all Jane's negative potentials into reverse and that within minutes she would be in the meditative state. I must point out at this stage that there is absolutely no danger to either the client's physical or mental health, provided the healer is competent and has a basic knowledge of psychology.

I was now behind Jane who was shaking violently, though apparently asleep. This state continued for about five minutes as I used all my spiritual and physical force-field to release a huge amount of pent-up passion which was about to explode from her. She told me afterwards that she felt it gather in her stomach and start to rise just like a gathering volcano. 'It was', she said, 'like a boiling rage of hate, something solid gathering inside me. I was sure', she went on, 'that the devil himself had entered my body and was going to explode inside.' As these emotions of hate and anger rose, so she began to shake even more violently until suddenly she let out a cry and I could physically feel a rush of energy leave her. The whole episode lasted about fifteen to twenty minutes.

What had taken place was a release of the emotions of anger and frustration which had been stored up ever since, as a little girl, Jane had been taught never to show anyone she was angry. So she grew to be an adult with the emotions of anger building in her body. This negative energy just kept growing. She had recently been through a pretty nasty divorce, and the jealousy, hate and other frustrations had added to the negative emotions already stored within her. She had become so completely consumed by anger that it was causing her physical pain, but because of her childhood conditioning it never showed itself in her disposition which was always loving. In anyone less emotionally strong it would have caused a nervous breakdown, depression or some other psychological trauma. If she had been less physically strong, this intense negative emotional energy might have caused the symptoms of multiple sclerosis, cancer, skin complaints or any one of a number of problems. As it was, she had contained this energy until now, when it had begun to escape to cause her pain. With the total release that the healing allowed, Jane was able to enjoy her life untroubled by further aches and pains. For the first time she was also able to find love in her heart for her parents, to forget the hurts of the past and look forward not backwards.

If what I had caused to happen had been witnessed 2000 years ago I would have been acclaimed for having exorcised the devil. If it had happened 250 years ago, or less they would have had me burnt at the stake for being the devil himself. As it is, more and more people come to me with emotional problems which are buried deep in their subconscious, but which none the less affect their peace of mind and quality of life. If left untreated, the effects of these long past traumas keep gate-crashing today's happiness.

In all of these sort of situations it's a matter of having the spiritual insight to read the client's symptoms, much as one would read a pictogram. Because the subconscious can't use words, it has to get its message across in pictures or actions. So all symptoms should be viewed as a message. It's a bit like doing a crossword puzzle. What would you think was the problem of a woman, aged thirty-nine, and exceptionally successful as a business manager? She was unmarried, and had no apparent social or personal problems, though she often suffered from business related stress. Her symptoms were excessive menstrual pain and a swelling abdomen. Her pain had been becoming more severe for several months and seemed to be directly linked to her distending stomach. At first the doctor thought it might be fibroids or a cyst, but internal examination proved it was neither of these. The uterus was many times larger than it should have been and the wall of the uterus hard and tight. The only action the hospital doctors could recommend was a hysterectomy.

At this point she asked if I could identify the cause of her condition. It seemed a straightforward enough situation but what I read in her symptoms seemed so improbable that at first I ignored it. However at a second interview I came to exactly the same conclusion. This was a phantom pregnancy. Her subconscious was desperately longing for a baby but material security and conscious logic had caused her to put the desire to the back of her thoughts. How could she have a baby and a career, she reasoned? Anyway she was not married and didn't have any relationship that could be considered suitable for raising a family.

Unfortunately the subconscious does not bother itself about small problems like logical reasoning. And because its charge was thirty-nine and just reaching an age where child-bearing would become unwise it had gone to the extreme lengths of producing the phantom pregnancy. The lady told me that she would love to have a baby, but it was quite impractical. While we were discussing the situation and her symptoms her distended abdomen, which for all the world looked as if she was about eight months pregnant, began to reduce in size. The subconscious had finally got its message through to its mistress's logical consciousness and could now absolve itself of all responsibility for reminding her that she needed to act quickly if she was going to have a baby.

I recall another lady who visited me because she had severe pains in her feet. She had been having medical treatment but the pain was so acute that walking was almost impossible. This was a classic psychosomatic disorder. I asked her how long she had had the problem and was told six years. I then asked what problem or trauma she had experienced six and a half years earlier. None she said.

Now one thing about being a healer is that if clients can't remember I can find out the information for myself because I contact the spiritual part of their consciousness. So I asked again. What happened six and a half years ago? Eventually I had to demand that she tell me. I could have told her what I knew, but I needed her to say it.

Eventually she admitted, though she could hardly bring herself to talk about it, that her husband had walked out on her six and a half years previously. This was a bitter humiliation. She had felt enormous anger and jealousy, but she assured me that this couldn't possibly be the reason for her troubled feet because she had remarried three years ago to a wonderful man and was very happy now and had put the past behind her.

I asked if she had ever cried about the break up of her first marriage and she said, certainly not. 'I wasn't going to let him think that he had hurt me.' At this point I went behind her and gave her conventional healing to completely relax her spirit and with that she broke down and sobbed for twenty minutes. When the time came to leave she walked to the door and said, 'All my pain has gone.' That was early 1990 and the pain in her feet has never returned.

Her subconscious was saying, you need to cry and talk about this to get rid of the hurt. Until you do the hurt will be in your feet. Why her feet? Well, that's another story.

Psychosomatic disorders have many causes. They can be a way of crying out for help, as in Tom's case, or an expression of hidden emotional trauma as in the cases just cited. The symptoms may be severe enough to cause anything from cramp to cancer.

Even heart problems can be psychosomatic. One such concerns a man, let's call him Brian, who had owned his own company. He had been very successful but the recession and financial pressures had put him under tremendous stress which had caused him to have a heart attack. He had recovered well, but it had left him very weak and unable to do any physical work. Even walking down the garden made him breathless and his heart pound.

What really annoyed him was the fact that the doctors had told him he was now physically well and the current problem was all due to stress. They said the recurring pain and physical symptoms were just psychosomatic. This he couldn't accept. A man doesn't cause his own heart attack and breathlessness, he told me. And when the doctors told him that he should see a psychiatrist he decided to finish with them and go to a healer. So that was the situation I was confronted with. I ran my hands over and through his electromagnetic field and could find nothing wrong with him whatsoever. I came to the same conclusion as the doctors which was that basically he had lost interest in his business and didn't want to tell his friends or colleagues that he was giving up. His subconscious had loyally provided an excuse. But how was I to tell him?

I let it go for a couple of weeks and after the first session he reported that he was feeling much better. In fact he said he had had a wonderful week. He had no pains and had been able to walk around the garden. The second week was not so good, he still felt better than before he first came to see me but he had made no improvement. The third week it was the same story. He started slipping back and by the fourth week he was nearly back to where he was when he first came to see me. Naturally he was disappointed that the early improvement had not been maintained. Now was my opportunity to confront him with the real problem.

'I'm not really surprised,' I said. 'You see, your subconscious has worked out how to beat me. It often happens, that when the subconscious is being over-protective of its charge it will eventually work out how to beat the system that is trying to help you. It wouldn't have mattered what treatment you were given, drugs or healing, eventually they would all have failed. It's not you, the sufferer, who is causing the problem, it's your subconscious.'

Does that mean I've got to see a psychiatrist?' he asked.

I told him I didn't think so because we had now identified the problem. It was obviously one of having to face his responsibilities at work. My advice was why fight it anyway? The whole problem regarding his health was directly connected with his job and it would be better to sell up or retire. He did this and a few months later he phoned to say his life had changed completely. He was now physically fit, especially since he had moved out of the area and the environment which was causing the problem.

REPRESSED CHILDHOOD TRAUMAS

One of the difficulties in explaining why symptoms are produced to identify trauma is why repress the trauma in the first place if our subconscious is going to produce health damaging symptoms to remind us as if playing some weird game of hide and seek. Most of the emotional and physical traumas which we repress happen before we reach eleven or twelve years of age. After that it has to be something pretty awful before the subconscious will take over and hide it from our conscious memory. Later in life, something happens which reminds the subconscious that a similar incident took place once before. To protect or warn us it then produces symptoms related to the past and the forgotten incident.

Emotional Traumas

We all accept that our basic character is formed in early childhood, the result of conditioning during our early years. Once we reach our teens, most of our emotions are already programmed into our character. Take, for instance, a child who is being regularly told to stop touching things. If he is told often enough he will grow up holding back and not wanting to experiment with new toys, games and eventually in a work situation, new methods.

I remember a parent asking me to help her son. Ted was eleven and had started at senior school just eight months earlier. He was having difficulty making friends. I asked him to explain his difficulties. For an eleven-year-old he was extremely articulate. He told me he had started very well at his new school. He had made some friends and become one of a group of six, all of whom he had known at his old school.

The problem had begun about three months later when a new lad had joined the group. He didn't know why but he felt threatened by this newcomer. I asked if this meant he was being bullied. That apparently wasn't the problem. In fact he liked the newcomer, who was fun to be with and always cracking jokes, fooling around and generally making people laugh. It was this which made him feel threatened. He didn't know why but he was sure that the other boys were not going to want him now. He couldn't explain it but this newcomer filled him with a feeling of loneliness and a feeling that he wasn't going to be wanted.

At this point I went behind him and placed my left hand over the centre of his forehead, i.e. between and above the eyes. This had the effect of inducing a changing state of consciousness, allowing strong emotion to surface from the past. While he was in this half asleep half awake state I asked him to recall the very first time he had felt the emotions he had just described. After a few seconds he told me that the earliest memory he had was when he was very young and his mother, father and sister were playing together in the living room (his sister is four years older than Ted). He felt left out as he wasn't allowed to join in or become involved. I asked why he hadn't gone across and joined in anyway.

'Oh I couldn't do that,' he said. 'I was only four weeks old.'

He then went on to recount another event. 'This time it was his sister's birthday party. With tears streaming down his face he told me how nobody had bothered about him while he lay in his cot in the corner. How he could hear all the laughter and fun but nobody paid him any attention or involved him in the games. On this occasion he was just a few months old.

A little later in his life he recalled how he had been in a carry-cot on the back seat of the car from where he could see nothing at all and how, when his father remarked about something in a field, they all laughed but nobody thought to tell him what was so funny or involve him in the situation. Still later he remembered being taken shopping and his mother promising to let the children choose their own toys. His sister, he said, was allowed to run about the shop and play with the toys on display and then choose one while he had to stay in the push-chair and his mother chose his toy.

'Could you walk?' I asked.

'No, but I could crawl,' he protested.

He went from one incident to the next, over a period of about twenty minutes until he got to the time when he was about twenty months old. He was walking now and feeling very pleased with himself, especially when his sister brought her friend into the garden to show off her brother's newfound ability to walk, but then the sister and friend went into the woods at the bottom of the garden. Again he wasn't allowed to go. He could hear them laughing and playing, but they didn't want him.

After this he must have started joining in because he had no further memories of being left out. So I removed my hand from the middle of his forehead and asked him how he felt. A big grin spread across his face.

'There's nothing wrong with my friends, is there? It's me.'

From that moment on he had no more trouble at school and he no longer feels that he's being 'left out' when there is laughter or fun. But think what would have happened if he hadn't come to see me to have his past revealed. He would have gone through his life withdrawing whenever there was the sound of laughter. He would have lost his ability to join in with excitement and happiness. His parents couldn't possibly have known what he was thinking or feeling at that early stage in his life, but their unwitting actions were laying the foundations for his attitudes and emotions later in life. Before Ted was two years old he had been conditioned to expect not to be included in activities associated with happiness and laughter.

Another case involving a young teenager illustrates just how careful adults have to be about making flippant remarks to, or in front of, young children who haven't yet developed an ability to know the difference between a serious comment and one made in fun.

I was asked to help a girl in her teens who had bed-wetting problems. Neither could she last very long during the day without going to the toilet and her condition bordered on incontinence. She had received all sorts of advice and treatment from doctors and psychologists, to no avail. She came with her mother who explained the problem. I asked her to close her eyes and then asked various questions about her childhood. As she went deeper into a changed state of consciousness I asked what had frightened her most as a young girl and she told me that when she was three she had been in hospital for a stomach operation and a nurse had come and told her to 'spend a penny or you will burst'. This short and seemingly innocent sentence had filled her with fear, the fear that if she didn't keep her bladder empty it would burst. It was now obvious why the subconscious was refusing to allow her bladder to hold water. Once the reason had been brought to logical consciousness her problem disappeared. But this illustrates how careful parents and other carers have to be about what they say in front of children.

I could fill another book just with the stories of people who have come to me for help because their lives have been ruined by the innocent actions of loving parents. I'll give one more example to illustrate the point.

A married woman in her fifties — let's call her Jill — came to me for help because she had no sense of self-worth. She always felt that any problems in her life were all her fault. If something had gone wrong then it must be her fault. Because she felt unworthy of love, she could find no enjoyment or pleasure in her sex life. This is such a problem for so many people.

Using the same technique, hand on a point above and between the eyes, I changed her state of consciousness and asked her to go back to the first time this had happened. Almost straight away she recalled walking home from school in the late autumn. She would have been about eight years old. She had to walk home from school along a quiet country lane. Suddenly a man came from behind and pushed her into the bushes where he sexually assaulted her. After about twenty minutes he let her go, warning her of what would happen if she should tell anyone.

By the time she got home it was quite late and getting dark. She ran into the kitchen to tell her mother what had happened. And as she started to blurt out her story, her mother, who was expecting some kind of excuse as a cover for being late, didn't let her daughter finish but snapped at her. 'And what time do you think this is? Coming home at this time of night is going to get you into trouble. All sorts of things can happen to a girl in a dark lane at night ... and you will have no one to blame but yourself ...'

After that, what could she do? It was her fault. A little girl of eight was condemned to spend the rest of her life feeling dirty and guilty because she knew that what had taken place was wrong and believed it was her fault. Hadn't her mother told her so? Her subconscious quickly repressed the memory of the ordeal but for ever after she would be conditioned to think that she was unworthy of love and affection, and if ever anything went wrong in her life after that she saw it as her fault. No blame can really be attached to the mother. But oh dear, the things we thoughtlessly say to our children that affect their emotions over a whole lifetime.

Fortunately it is never too late to rid yourself of the restricting conditioning imposed on you in childhood. Conditioning of this kind usually takes place before the age of eleven, after which we seem to be able to reason independently and the subconscious becomes less able to repress the memory of uncomfortable situations. Even adults, though, can find that complete sequences of their lives have been 'lost' to memory if recalling them is too painful to bear. I suppose car accidents are the most obvious examples of such traumas.

Physical Traumas

The cases I've just described show how attitudes and emotions can be affected by early trauma. The following case histories are examples of how a trauma in early childhood can cause physical symptoms.

Eczema and psoriasis are skin conditions in which very sore patches appear on the surface of the body and I have had more than one case which has been the direct result of a childhood beating. In one case a woman had psoriasis on her legs and arms where she had been abused by bullies at school. In another case a man had psoriasis patches over his body where he had been beaten as a child by his father. Neither of the victims remembered the incidents until treatment began and in both cases the psoriasis began to fade once the reason for it was acknowledged. Also, in both cases, the condition did not appear until their late teens when the subconscious was given reason to believe that a similar situation might occur again.

This does not mean that all cases of eczema or psoriasis are the direct result of childhood abuse. It's just that sometimes they are. There can be dozens of reasons for skin reactions. Other cases of eczema I have had involved the hands. One of the people had had a series of accidents and problems, from babyhood to adulthood, all involving her hands. The problems included being burnt, stung, slapped etc. When she got married and had her own children, her subconscious was prompted to recall details of her own childhood and this resulted in blistering hands. Another involved someone whose hands became terribly sore and painful when he went into building work. It all began when he went to demolish a building in which he had found happiness as a child when life at home was not so happy. His subconscious just wouldn't allow him to pull down the building which had been his refuge as a child. The result was blistering hands which were diagnosed as a reaction to the lime mortar that held the old building together.

Birth Traumas

It's surprising how many people come for help with depression or a feeling of panic which is the result of a birth trauma. From my experience it would seem that some cases of post-natal depression are caused by the mother having experienced a very difficult and frightening time at the moment of her own birth. Then, like all other childhood traumas it was repressed by the over-protective subconscious, which let it resurface at the time she gave birth to her own children.

This is especially true if the mother had labour problems which were similar to her own mother's labour problems. As the mother is giving birth to her own children, so the subconscious partially releases the memory of her own trauma and emotion all those years ago when she herself was being born. The problem then is that, once partially released, the trauma cannot be repressed again. And so the mother continues for days, weeks, months or even years to be plagued by feelings of panic, breathlessness and tearfulness which are collectively termed depression or stress.

Recently a woman came to me suffering, as she put it, from stress. She explained that she had been having palpitations and so her doctor had put her on to beta-blockers. She was very emotional and could easily break down and cry. She also had periods of breathlessness and generally felt run down and out of sorts. I could see that this was going to be relatively easily resolved so, without explanation, I stood behind her and began a normal healing session, i.e. hands over the top of the head. I could feel the power flowing from me into her.

She immediately became breathless. Her breathing was fast and shallow, her heart was pumping like fury and she started to tense up. After about five minutes she let out a scream followed by a series of short, sharp cries and then several long screams. Then she just sobbed and gasped as if she was almost choking. I let her get it all out of her system, which must have taken fifteen minutes. When I was sure all the emotion had passed I stopped the healing.

'What on earth was that?' she asked.

'Did you have a difficult birth?'

'Yes,' she answered. 'Apparently I almost died. For some reason I was positioned feet first and wouldn't come out.'

'Well, you have just gone through it all again,' I said. 'That was a birth trauma and all the symptoms you've been experiencing were your emotions of panic as you were being born. What I want to know is, what has triggered it now? Have you recently had a baby?'

She then went on to tell me that she had had a baby girl three and a half years earlier who had been born exactly the same way she had. It had been an awful experience, she said. So that was it. Giving birth to her daughter had partially released her own birth trauma. The symptoms had continued for the next three and a half years and they were diagnosed first as post-natal depression and then as depression. The symptoms would have persisted for the rest of her life if she hadn't done something about having them released.

'How do you feel now?' I asked, though it wasn't really necessary to enquire. I could see by the expression on her face how elated she was. Gone were the drawn, tired, frightened features. She positively glowed with happiness.

'I don't believe it's possible,' she said. 'In less than half an hour I feel as if I've been reborn. I feel wonderful, fantastic.'

There is another point here which is worth noting, and that is the terror which is sometimes experienced by the baby while it is being born. It isn't only the mother who suffers during a difficult birth. The baby can also have a terrible time and unfortunately, unlike the mother who usually recovers fairly quickly from the ordeal, the baby's trauma might affect the rest of its life. Some thought should therefore be given to the conversations which the baby might hear from within the mother's womb. Talk of difficult births, caesarian births, etc. must strike panic into an unborn child. If it becomes necessary to talk of birth I suggest that the pregnant mother talks to her baby and puts its mind at rest.

It must also be very distressing for the unborn baby if its parents are desperate for a girl and it's a boy they are going to get, especially if they keep telling everyone that they are sure it will be a girl. The poor child is going to feel rejected before it's born. This sense of rejection will become part of its character which it will use for subconscious decision-making later in life. A lot of people may not believe that an unborn baby can hear and form judgements and experience emotions before being born. But hardly a week goes by that I don't encounter a person whose character was formed by extreme emotions before their birth. I've always maintained that, compared with being born, dying is easy.

───── *PSYCHOSOMATIC PAIN* ─────

Psychosomatic pain is a term used to describe pain or discomfort when there is no apparent illness or injury which could be causing it. I have separated psychosomatic pain into three separate categories. The first is habitual. This is when the pain continues long after the reason for it has passed. This usually happens when the pain has been intense for long periods of time. The second is when the original cause of the pain was so horrific that the subconscious warns and reminds the victim of the event if he looks like involving himself in a similar situation. And the third is where the emotions at the time of the original pain were ones of intense fear, guilt or passion of some other sort.

In the first two cases it is often only necessary to make a logical, conscious connection between the current pain and the problem which caused the initial injury to cure it. The third category is not so simply dealt with, though. Because deep, repressed emotions are involved, it requires more time and understanding of subconscious behaviour and recall to overcome the difficulties. As always, I will try to illustrate this using actual cases.

Habitual Pain

When pain has been very intense for a long time, and the cause of the pain is eventually dealt with, the brain sometimes fails to register the fact and the sufferer continues to feel pain even though all reason for it has gone.

Doctors and healers are often blamed simply because they cannot rid the sufferer of a pain which the brain has forgotten to switch off. I remember one particular case of a man who had had several operations on his knee to try and deal with a pain which the doctors said didn't exist. The patient was annoyed at not being believed and the doctors thought he was making it up, when all the time it was the fault of a sticky switch called habit, in the brain.

The brain is programmed to act in a given way and it will continue to do so without any help from consciousness. As an example, lets say the indicators in your car are on the left of the steering wheel and the windscreen wipers on the right. Now imagine getting into a car with these two controls reversed. How often do you indicate with the windscreen wipers? This is a habit, a program in the brain which hasn't yet been updated. It's a bit inconvenient for a day or two but you get the brain recoded and all returns to normal. But what happens when you don't realise that the problem is in the brain's program?

John was twenty-eight, very fit and athletic. His particular problem was a pain in his left knee, just below the kneecap. After two healing sessions and no improvement I realised that I had to look for a cause other than an injury. His knee was hurting most of the time, but didn't seem to interfere too much with his sports except that he couldn't run more than a mile at a time. That sounded just a bit too precise to my way of thinking and was just the sort of key to the cause of his problem that I was looking for.

'So it always starts to really hurt when you've run just a mile, does it?' I questioned.

'Always,' he said. 'I can run a mile without more than the

usual pain, but a mile is just that bit too far.'

Then I got the full story. He had been keeping fit by jogging and increasing his distance each week. He had wanted to run in a marathon somewhere and was doing his training on his local athletics track. One evening, when he had run 8 miles (note the precision again) around the track his knee suddenly gave in. I'm not too sure what actually happened but something went wrong with the ligaments which resulted in a pain below the knee-cap. Apparently it was an excruciating pain which needed a lot of treatment and time in hospital. Months later he had been declared totally fit but his knee continued to give him this constant pain.

'It's just like toothache,' he said 'and when I've run a mile it gets really bad.'

'How do you know it's exactly a mile when the excruciating pain starts?'

'Because there's a mile sign on the track.'

'How did you know you had gone exactly 8 miles when the knee let you down the first time?'

'Because I had just reached the mile marker for the eighth time.' I think I heard him mutter under his breath at that question.

'The only thing that's wrong with you,' I said, 'is that your brain needs reprogramming.'

I then went on to explain that it had become so important to him to complete a given number of laps that the mile marker had become fixed in his mind. He had been concentrating so intensely on the distance that, when he passed the mile marker and his knee gave in, the brain recorded the mile as well as the pain and put it into the program. The mile became part of the habit. There was nothing wrong with his knee now. The pain he was experiencing was entirely due to his habitual running routine and going past the 1 mile marker. All it took was to register in his logical mind what the subconscious was trying to tell him. I used suggestive therapy to ensure the pain habit was removed and he was quickly back to normal.

This is a typical case of physical pain being caused by the brain's computer building the experience of pain into it's program. It's quite easy to deal with once it's been diagnosed and healers are far more able to help people with these problems if they know how to recognise the symptoms or read the deeper thoughts of their clients. Doctors don't have a chance of understanding, diagnosing or curing the sort of problems I've just been describing. They often see as many patients a day as I see in five days. And no matter how brilliant the doctor, or how caring, it's time that people need most. Unfortunately that's usually the one thing a doctor can't spare.

Warning Pain

The following story illustrates the difference between habitual pain and pain created by a subconscious wanting to warn it's body to avoid possible pain, based on previous experience.

A woman of thirty-two came to me in March with backache. She explained that she had been having pain in her lower back since she was about twenty. Her doctor thought it was a damaged disc which was affected by cold winter weather. Apparently the pains went once the weather warmed up in spring, but always returned again in late winter. The pain was so acute that the only place she could sleep was on the floor. I asked if she had any children. She told me she had a fourteen-year-old boy. I then asked which month he was born in.

She gave me a questioning look and said, 'Late February, why?'

Ignoring her question, I went on. 'Where were you lying when your baby was born?'

'I was on a bed.'

'And was it a difficult birth?'

'A very difficult one,' she replied. By now her voice was trailing off, as the significance of what I was saying began to take hold. For fourteen years her subconscious had been warning her every February to take care and remember what happened that February fourteen years ago when she lay on a bed. Is it any wonder that her subconscious wouldn't give her any peace in February, especially, when she went to lie down on a bed? All this took fifteen minutes to explain. At this point I asked her to stand up, walk round and touch her toes, all of which she did, though she hadn't been able to fifteen minutes earlier. Her subconscious had now given up responsibility for protecting her, as the symptoms it had so faithfully been producing had been understood. Her pain had been completely removed in just fifteen minutes and I didn't even have to get up from my chair.

As we have seen, the subconscious will sometimes create symptoms to avoid pain it thinks is going to happen, based on previous experience. Why people go skiing I shall never know. To slide around on two pieces of polished wood in freezing conditions at great risk of breaking or twisting some part of your anatomy, is completely beyond me. It would make more sense if it was free but it is so expensive.

I know at least one person who now thinks as I do. On the first morning of his first skiing holiday he was up on the slopes in Switzerland by 9 a.m. By lunchtime he was back in his hotel with his leg in plaster. He had broken his tibia just above the ankle. He told me that he had only been standing on the slopes for about fifteen minutes when he broke his leg. He was listening to the ski instructor giving some advice. After a while he was asked to move forward, but somehow his skis had crossed and over he went. He said the pain was indescribable. He really thought he had ripped his foot off. He had never known pain like it.

This had all happened several years ago and everything had apparently healed well. The problem now was that the left leg, the injured one, kept going numb from the waist down to his toes. 'It just goes totally dead!' was how he described it. He hadn't associated this with his skiing injury. Why should he? That had healed completely. Like the doctors, he thought it must be something to do with a trapped nerve in his back. The

103

reason he was so concerned about his leg was because he was liable to fall and his job required him to be on his feet a lot. He was all right so long as he kept moving but if he stood still his leg soon went numb. Could I do anything?

During the first session I went over his back with my hands but couldn't find anything wrong. So the following week I asked him if he had ever had an accident, which is when I got all the details of the skiing injury. Two things stuck in my mind. One was that he had only been on the slopes fifteen minutes when his accident happened. The other was that if he stood still for about ten minutes his leg went numb. So I asked him to check, during the coming week, exactly how long he had to stand still before his leg went numb. He reported back the following week that it was twelve minutes each time.

Now I put it to him that his accident had happened about thirteen minutes after he had gone on to the slopes and the pain had been so terrible that his subconscious had noted in great detail exactly how long it was after he had been standing that this awful pain had started. To ensure that there was no repetition of such an excruciating pain, every time he stood for twelve minutes his subconscious took over and cut off all sensation to that leg. In fact there was nothing wrong with his leg; it was just his subconscious being over-protective. Once the subconscious had got its message across to his logical consciousness it gave up its responsibility for controlling the time he stood on the leg and the leg never gave any more problems. So healing is also about being in tune with another's deeper thoughts and using your intuition to decode their symptoms.

Trauma Pain

As I have explained, psychosomatic pain can also be the symptom of a trauma, though a healer needs to have mental awareness and deep spiritual insight to recognise this.

The first time I recall realising that pain was a symptom of a trauma was at a talk I was giving. It had gone quite well and the expected one hour's discussion had become three.

At the end of the meeting a lady came up to me and asked if I would do something about her back pain. She must have been about thirty-five and was obviously suffering acute pain roughly halfway down her back. I placed my hands on the area of pain and she immediately began to bend forward. Then she twisted and bent backwards, all quite involuntarily. After about fifteen minutes her body went limp and she said all the pain had gone. It was October and I just knew she would be visiting me at the same time next year. So I gave her my card and said, 'If you ever need me again make an appointment.' I heard nothing more from her until the following September. She came with her husband and explained that she hadn't had any back pain at all since I had given her treatment the previous October but in the last week it had come back again. So I asked her to sit down and this time, while I was treating her back, I explained what was causing the pain.

First I asked if the pain came on every autumn. She agreed that it did. Furthermore it seemed to persist all winter and then go in the spring and it had been like that for years. It was obvious that she must have had an accident as a little girl, that it must have been in the autumn when the leaves were changing colour, and that the accident — though probably not serious in itself — had created a terrible sense of fear in her mind. After the incident, or whatever it was, her subconscious had repressed her conscious memory of it but each autumn, when the leaves changed colour, her subconscious reacted by sending out warning signals of impending danger. It did this by causing back pain.

She was quite incredulous, said she loved autumn colours and couldn't remember anything that had frightened her. But she promised to check with her father when she got home, her mother having since died. She phoned back a few hours later with the full story which her father had remembered in detail. When she was two or three years old the family had visited Windsor Castle and her father had stood her on the parapet so that she could see the view more clearly, which was beautiful because of the golden colour of the autumn foliage. Just for a second, her father had turned around to say something to her mother and loosened his grip on her hand. At that moment she had stumbled and slipped over the edge of the wall.

Acting on instinct, her father had grabbed hold of whatever came into his fingers as she disappeared over the edge. He caught hold of her hair and coat collar and hauled her back on to the top. She had gone as white as a ghost. I don't expect her father looked too good either, probably green, and she had also lost her voice. She was taken to see the doctor who advised that they say nothing about the incident, and hopefully as the incident and the fear were forgotten her voice would return, which it did several days later.

But the memory of it all still remained in her subconscious to remind her to be careful each autumn when the leaves were turning gold. The pain was her subconscious saying autumn is here, be careful. The back pain must have been caused at the time of the fall, though any physical injury had long since gone. Fortunately she had always resisted surgery, which would have served no useful purpose and certainly wouldn't have got rid of pyschosomatic pain. Once the incident had been brought to logical consciousness, she had no further trouble.

Another point must be understood here. If there had been some emotional trauma involved, based on guilt, even if the guilt was wrongly perceived, then it would not have been quite so easy to cure the problem. This sort of straightforward healing only works when the problem is purely physical. If guilt or some other fear-based emotion had been involved then it would have been necessary to cause the client to experience the event as a physical, emotional or memory recall. Healing would then have automatically released the repressed details if it had been necessary, though it might have taken several sessions to do so.

CANCER

I suppose of all health problems the one most people dread is cancer, for two main reasons. Firstly, it is invariably thought to be terminal and secondly, the distressing symptoms which the dying have to endure have caused the word itself to become taboo. This doesn't help at all, as very often the cancer is caused by an emotional problem or trauma which is also not discussed, especially as it's not usual to associate past difficulties in life with current health problems. I find that when I explain to a client what is going on and how we are going to beat it they immediately start to relax. Not knowing is the biggest cause of fear and fear creates pain.

Cancer does not normally arise from a disease or an inherited genetic disorder but from a normal cell in the body reverting to a primitive state, or more correctly not developing to become a specialised cell such as a liver cell or a blood cell. This in itself should not be a problem. The odd cell, one out of millions, having no special feature to give it a reason for being, is usually dealt with by the body's own defence system. But sometimes the body lets such cells grow, and the simpler the cell type the faster they will multiply and the harder they are to treat. The subconscious uses these unspecialised cells to produce symptoms of distress.

A tumour is different from a cancer because a tumour cell is not unlike the cell it originated from. It retains its speciality and is therefore slower to multiply, easier to deal with and less likely to wander off to some other part of the body. Cancer cells, being very simple and basic, multiply so rapidly and wildly that they require far more of the body's nutrients to keep pace with their growth than are required by the carefully controlled multiplication of normal cells. Also, the wild, uncontrolled expansion of cancer cells means that they don't care how much of the body they move into and take over. They spread so rapidly that, if left untreated, they starve the body of all nutrients, causing it to wither and die.

A doctor's view of how cancer should be treated is different from that of a healer. The doctor, with all the weapons of war at his disposal, prefers the 'aggressive' approach. He believes that the only way to deal with cancer is to cut it out with surgery, poison it with drugs or blast it with x-rays. But after sixty years or more doctors still haven't won this war or got anywhere near to beating cancer. And sometimes the treatment does more harm than enemy. Healers can't claim to have made any great breakthroughs either, though our successes are probably on a par with orthodox medicine, but at least we don't add to the pain and humiliation the disease causes.

Healers fight this problem with the help of the patient. Unlike orthodox medicine, which considers the patient's involvement almost an intrusion into affairs which don't concern them, healers cannot begin their work without the co-operation of the patient. The patient, the spirit within the body, is the one who is going to win or lose this battle. He or she is the one with the most to lose or to gain. Therefore, as the patients are in direct communication with this hyped-up, idiotic army of cells, they are the ones who are going to have to confront it, communicate with it, dissuade it from advancing further and eventually persuade it to once again revert to type and become a specialised cell. To do this, they have to communicate with the army commander, the subconscious. The healer aids, guides and gives strength to the client so that he can once again resume full control of his own body.

Of course a lot depends on exactly what the initial cause was which prompted the cell to 'go it alone', and here we come back to psychosomatic symptoms. It is the cause which has to be overcome, not the symptoms. I am sure that many of the causes of cancer begin with a trauma. I remember vividly a woman who willed herself to die of cancer because her husband had left her. She was convinced that once she had cancer he would return to her. Her cancer developed after he left and she told me quite candidly that she had nothing to live for, unless her husband returned. Unfortunately he didn't, and no treatment, orthodox or otherwise, made the slightest difference to her condition. Healing did remove her pain, physical pain that is, but nothing could reach the pain in her soul.

I treat many cancer patients every year and I don't claim to have worked any miracles, though in most cases I can help relieve pain. Patients are then able to pass from their bodies into a more peaceful world free of the fear and terrible humiliation which a drug-soaked body suffers.

Cancers caused by emotional trauma or negative attitudes are difficult to deal with. As a healer the best I can hope for, until the cause of the trauma is identified, is to ease the pain and fear and create a sense of calm in the client. Unless the hidden emotional trauma can be identified and brought from subconscious to logical consciousness, one can only achieve a holding situation in which the client, with regular treatment, neither improves nor gets worse. Until the inner emotional conflict can be settled there is little likelihood of a cure.

Lack of Self-worth

A woman in her late forties came for treatment. She had already had a mastectomy three years before and now she had secondaries. The problem had spread to, or started anew, in her lungs. Like most people in her condition, she had lost a lot of weight due to the malignant cells having an insatiable appetite and starving the rest of the body.

In these situations I always recommend that the patient immediately goes on to high doses of vitamin C-rich glucose, at about 5 dessertspoons a day. The reason for taking glucose is simply that, unless energy can be provided in excess of what the cancer cells take, the body loses its strength and ability to fight. I also recommend the vitamin C because there is some evidence that large doses of vitamin C slow the growth of malignant cells. Anything which can do this, and is neither addictive nor a harmful chemical, must be a valuable aid.

Incidentally I should like to stress at this point that I refuse to take patients who are not under the supervision of a doctor or who decline to tell their doctor that they are visiting me and what I am doing. I am fortunate that so many doctors recommend me to their patients.

To return to the lady with lung cancer, her problem was an emotional one. She had been brought up in a strictly religious household where sex outside marriage was strictly forbidden. To enforce obedience, her religion warned that extra-marital relationships would be opposed by God and anyone who strayed would be forever damned.

Unfortunately this woman had not contracted a good marriage and in a moment of need had many years before formed a deep emotional and physical attachment to another man. This continued in secret for a year or so. Eventually whatever it was that had caused her to seek love outside her marriage was overcome and she went on for many years with a happy marriage. However the thoughts of that earlier transgression began to haunt her more and more until she was racked with guilt.

She was sure she had sinned. Even though, to some extent, I was able to convince her that she was in no way damned or forgotten by God, she could not overcome the thought that she had sinned against her own integrity. This was the cause of her cancer; she was, subconsciously, actively disfiguring herself. She had been a beautiful woman who now thought of herself because of her transgression, as ugly. No amount of talk or persuasion, no amount of love or healing, would distract this woman from destroying herself through guilt.

I see many cases of breast cancer every year and nearly all the women concerned have one thing in common — a lack of self-worth, a feeling of having lost their reason for being. With some it's because they've retired from a job they've held for many years. With others it's because their children have grown up and don't need their mother any more. Their husbands are fully involved in a separate social life or a busy working life, leaving the mother feeling as if her usefulness to the family is finished. The symptoms of breast cancer then become an unrealised cry for a purpose in life. Unless the cause is found and dealt with the subconscious often continues its battle for attention by producing secondaries. With others it's because they have moved away from their mother or father and feel guilty about leaving them.

Only recently a woman came to me who many years earlier had had a mastectomy. Then the cancer appeared in the remaining breast which resulted in another mastectomy. Her subconscious then started to produce secondaries in her lungs and bones. At this point I was asked to help. On her second visit we had a long discussion and it transpired that just before the first breast cancer she had recently moved to another part of the country, away from her parents. She felt particularly unhappy about this, but her husband's work demanded that they move. The cancer appeared for the second time immediately before her twenty-year-old daughter left home to go abroad. Now she seemed to have lost everything. This time her subconscious would not be deprived.

The point had been reached where the doctors could do no more. When I explained, and she became aware of her part in the cancer's appearance, and that all was not lost, she immediately began to improve. Time will tell if she has truly come to terms with her new situation. But as she said, 'Above everything else you have made me realise that there is hope. I am my own cure.'

I have had many successes with people who have come to me with cancers when all seemed lost and they all say the same, 'You gave me hope when there was none by giving me a reason for it all.'

Fear

Of course, not all breast cancers are caused by a feeling of rejection, or worthlessness. I remember one young woman who had had a lumpectomy (i.e. the removal of a cancerous lump from the breast). All seemed to have gone well and there was no reason to suppose that she would have any more problems. But quite soon after treatment cancerous cells were found in the lymph glands. The doctors could give no reason for this especially as she was only twenty-eight, getting married in a few months' time and seemingly had everything to live for.

However, her deeper emotions eventually surfaced, as they so often do in spiritual healing sessions. She told me she had been living with her boyfriend for many years and that he had wanted to marry her from the start. She had refused to marry at first because they needed time to be sure, then she delayed the wedding again because of the need to save to buy a house, and she kept coming up with one excuse after another to postpone the wedding. The real reason she felt, though she hadn't considered it before, was that she wouldn't be able to manage the extra responsibility. But on deeper investigation it transpired that what was really frightening her was the idea of having to be responsible for a family.

The thought of having children scared her so much that when her subconscious realised the wedding couldn't be put off any longer it had provided a further excuse for delaying the marriage: cancer. Because the fear was related to children and nurturing, so it produced its message of fear in the breast. The doctors had dealt with the physical symptoms by surgical means, but they hadn't done anything about the cause. So the subconscious just created another set of symptoms by producing more cancer cells, this time in the lymph glands of the same breast. The doctors could have gone on treating the symptoms for as long as the body could stand it, but the subconscious would have continued trying to get its message across and would have gone on producing secondary cancers, until its message was decoded and recognised.

As soon as she realised that her unspoken fears were the cause of her cancer the problem disappeared. The marriage was postponed, but only until her fear of having and being responsible for children was sorted out.

Fatalism

Another interesting case concerned a man in his mid-forties. He had been diagnosed as having lung cancer some twelve months before he came to see me. He came, like so many others, not so much because he believed in healing but because there was nowhere else to go for help. The medical profession had done all they could and for some reason he could have no more chemotherapy or radiotherapy. He had been told he might have about three months left. He came more because his wife insisted than out of a belief that healing might help.

I never did discover the original cause of his cancer but one thing was certain: unless I could persuade him that he could live beyond three months the doctor's prophecy would be fulfilled. It took a few weeks to get to know him intimately and during that time I sustained him with the usual glucose and healing energies. When I had all the information about his life that I needed I began. My whole aim was to change his attitude. We will call him John and the dialogue, considerably edited, went something like this:

'You weren't very clever when you were young, were you John?'

'No, not really,' he replied.

He agreed that his parents hadn't expected him to achieve much at school, and so he hadn't disappointed them.

Again, when he started work no one expected him to amount to much, and so no one was surprised when he didn't do well. All his life he had done just as everyone had predicted. His problem was that he didn't like disappointing people, or making waves. So again, it hadn't surprised anyone when he'd caused his family their present problems by becoming ill.

At this point I decided to confront him directly.

'In fact, John,' I said, 'you prefer to agree with people so much, in preference to argument, that you will even agree with the doctors when they say you will die in another ten weeks. Correct?'

113

There was a long pause, and then he said, 'I'm not going to make some .... Doctor happy by dying for him.'

I challenged him again. 'But that's what they expect you to do and you always do what's expected of you.'

Finally John answered, with anger rising in his voice. 'Then I'm going to have to upset a few people because I'm not going to die to please anyone.'

John's cancer regressed and he was well and happy for a further two years. Then he had an emotional shock which was unconnected with his family and the cancer returned. This time he was unable to respond with the will to live.

As he and many others have said to me, 'The thing you did more than anything else was make me realise I could beat it. That my body and its maintenance was under my control.' Unfortunately the medical profession are not trained to think in this way. They think the body is under *their* control and when they fail they leave their victims believing that nothing else can be done.

Positive Results

As I have said before, only some cancers are emotionally caused. But a lot of suffering could be avoided if some thought was given to treatment of underlying trauma before embarking on sophisticated chemical and surgical technology as a form of cure.

Even those cancers which don't appear to have an emotional cause will often respond very well to a simple laying on of hands without any medical help. One such case was a lady who asked if I could help with a cancerous growth on the top of her head. It had been forming for several months and when she came to me it was 1.5 to 2 centimetres across and protruded about 1 centimetre above her scalp.

Normally I will only treat clients with problems such as cancer if they are already seeing a doctor or agree to see one immediately after visiting me. However this particular lady had a phobia about doctors, or rather cancer and doctors, and so I agreed to see her on three consecutive days for half an hour on each visit. There didn't seem to be any need for discussion, so I went straight into healing by holding the centre fingers of my left hand just above the cancerous tissue. Each healing lasted about twenty minutes.

On the morning after the third visit she phoned to tell me that the offending tissue had fallen out that morning. I saw her once more and could see that there was nothing left except a small hollow where the cancer had been. Within a few months the site returned to normal. I have treated several skin cancers and most of these have responded exceptionally well to healing.

It is very rare to cure internal cancers. But there are those who, through great personal courage and determination, confuse all the laws of medicine and biology. One such was a lady in her seventies whom I recall very clearly. She came to me with her doctor's blessing. Her cancer was in the stomach and it was decided that nothing further could be done. From the day she began to visit, once a week, she never again suffered pain and refused all the pain killers offered, stating quite categorically that she hadn't any pain.

She first visited me in October and her cancer was clearly at an advanced stage. It wasn't thought she would live beyond Christmas. We talked about life and how one moves from this world to the next and I told her, as I tell everyone who comes to me for help, I don't make any promises. But she did wring one promise from me — which was that I would keep her going until after her grand-daughter's wedding, which was planned for September of the following year, still ten months away.

Well, she kept going and, without the aid of sticks, she appeared in the photographs of her grand-daughter's wedding. A week or two later she went into hospital and, on the second night there, passed peacefully away. No fear, no pain, no drugs.

— 6 —

Programming

Most of you by now will have realised that there is a strong element of hypnosis in healing. However, very few healers I have ever spoken to would admit this. They prefer some deeper mystical or spiritual meaning to it all. Although there is a deeper spiritual side to healing, it must be faced that healers and hypnotists, or rather hypno-analysts have a lot in common. The only difference between them is that one knows it and the other doesn't. The hypnotist stays mostly in the realm of emotional problems, not having given much thought to his ability as a healer. And the healer, feeling demeaned if someone should suggest he's probably using hypnosis, refuses to accept the benefits which would come to his aid if he wasn't so high-brow.

Franz Anton Mesmer, born in 1734 in Austria, gave the world mesmerism, the forerunner of the more complex art of hypnosis. Mesmer believed in many of the things mentioned in this book. In a way he was also an early healer. He used sweeping passes of his hands, just as many healers do, though he never used the term spiritual. To him all healing was of a physical or mental origin and it was Mesmer who first added the phrase 'animal magnetism' to the world of medicine.

116

Although he had two doctorates, in medicine and philosophy, his colleagues were hostile to most of his claims. (Not much has changed in the 250 years since his birth; and scientists and academics still tend to be very sceptical.) Mesmer believed that there was a bio-magnetic field around the body, and using magnets he was able to demonstrate a remarkable list of cures, including epilepsy, hysteria and depression. His method was to apply horseshoe magnets to the patient's body, the soles of their feet and on their chest. He believed that there was a magnetic field around the body and interference with this flow could harm or improve mental or physical health. Disheartened because of criticism by his own profession, who used the fact that he couldn't cure a blind girl with magnets as proof of quackery, he decided to leave for Paris.

In Paris he utilised a contraption which was basically a tub in which the water had been magnetised. People would sit around the tub holding hands while Mesmer walked around passing his hands over them and fixing others with his penetrating eyes — probably the first example of group therapy. This was in the 1780s, long before the modern theories of biochemistry or biophysics had become known. Even so, if we compare his practices with modern healing methods and electromagnetic field theories we have to concede that maybe he wasn't so far off the mark.

His success was so great that he eventually took to treating up to 100 people at a time in a strange sort of group therapy which involved those taking part having to hold a cord attached to a tree. Many of these people subsequently reported their conditions as having been cured or much improved. He went on to found the Society of Harmony (an inspired precursor to the Holistic Medical Association which was to be formed 200 years later). But the orthodox medical profession gave him no quarter and anyone associated with him, or in later years his theories, was likely to be expelled from the medical profession. This short-sighted approach probably held healing back by 200 years.

Only in recent times has healing come to be accepted for what it is, an opportunity for the populace at large to help each other to better health. In the laying on of hands the practitioner is influencing the electromagnetic field around the one he is treating. There is absolutely no doubt about this. We are all affected by or affect those with whom we come into close contact. If our powers of thought are strong enough or if there is already a harmonising bond, we can affect others at a great distance from us. If any idea has merit and is of value to society then eventually, no matter what opponents with vested interests may say or do, it will succeed. This has been the case with healing and many other therapies.

So, what is the hypnotic state? No one can really be sure except to say that for some reason the logical, conscious mind becomes inactive, allowing suggestions to be received and programmed into the subconscious mind without being sub-jected to critical analysis first. Whatever is suggested to the subconscious, which is not being guarded by a reasoning and logical waking consciousness, will be received, accepted without question, recorded and acted on if the situation demands it. The hypnotic state is induced when someone with a strong electro-magnetic field neutralises the field of another who allows it, thus suspending the usual logical reasoning processes.

In his book, *The Body Electric*, Dr Robert O. Becker tells of an American doctor who uses hypnosis to control pain in his patients and who has shown that the frontal, negative potentials of the head become less negative as the patient goes deeper into trance. In fact, he goes on, the potential can drop to zero if the reversed current is strong enough. Interestingly, this is exactly what happens in anaesthesia. So, in essence, there is little difference between hypnotic anaesthesia and chemical anaes-thesia. In both situations negative potentials at the extremities weaken or vanish as anaesthesia takes effect. Under deep anaesthesia they reverse entirely.

Dr Becker tells us that when the American doctor gave the suggestion for pain control in the arm, the potential of that arm reversed, exactly as it had in response to a procain injection. He also found that when the patient was in an awakened state concentration on the arm increased the pain as the potential became more negative. He says this shows quite clearly that hypnosis actually blocks the pain and doesn't just prevent the patient from responding to it. It shows that the brain can cut off pain by altering the direct current potentials of the body.

Suggestibility

Now I know all this sounds highly technical and this isn't supposed to be a technical book. But I do think it's important to point out the similarities between the hypnotic state, healing and chemical anaesthesia. All these produce identical altered brain potentials. This should be very carefully kept in mind by those working within earshot of patients under anaesthetic or in a healing state.

The hypnotist is well aware that anything he says to his hypnotised patient will be uncritically accepted by the subconscious and acted on, but others in the caring professions do not always realise this. Careless talk in the operating theatre or healing room, before the patient has recovered, can do untold damage. Anaesthetised patients will act on information subconsciously heard. So it should always be assumed, even though the patient appears to be asleep or day-dreaming that the subconscious is registering literally everything it hears. For this reason the only comments that should be made while healing or caring for a patient should be positive ones. This is an important way of adding positive suggestibility to a patient's self-healing potential.

What of healers? They are well aware, or should be, that they are influencing the electromagnetic field of their client. But I believe that many don't know how they are doing it or what sort of effect their own stronger field will have upon the one they are helping. I see healers putting their hands around the foreheads of clients and the clients going into a state of deep relaxation. Anyone who has received healing will tell you how wonderfully relaxing it is. It is well known that those who have faith, i.e. expect to benefit from healing, will feel a positive benefit. Those who don't, won't.

This is not what is known as a 'psychological benefit'. The benefit gained is very real, because during the healing session the healer actually reduces the direct current through the client's brain, producing a changed-state consciousness (the state reached just before we go to sleep). The healer is unwittingly inducing a hypnotic state in which the client, who is expecting his pain to ease or some other physical or emotional problem to improve, actually creates his own suggestion therapy. The healer helps the client to enter into a state of mild, sometimes deep hypnosis, and the client then feeds directly into his own subconscious, his own expectations and hopes.

It's the most natural, basic and beneficial type of health treatment I know, provided the healer doesn't offer comments or advice while his client is in any level of the hypnotic state. I once heard a healer say to a client as he was coming out of the healing state, 'You will probably have trouble with that hand for the rest of your life.' He will now! The client's subconscious will certainly act on a suggestion so positively put. But I've known doctors say things even more crass to patients who have been in a state of shock, such as at the moment they are told they have cancer, or when they are recovering from an operation.

I've heard healers say to clients they are treating, 'It will probably hurt for a day or two, but you should be all right by Tuesday.' And guess what? The client will report back that the healer was absolutely right. They had pain until going to bed on the Monday, but it had all gone by Tuesday. How did the healer know? The healer didn't know. He just implanted the suggestion without realising it. The fact that he said it caused him to be proved correct. I know because I've done it myself, in order to test the theory. I've made comments like, 'You will have no pain except on next Thursday, four days from now when it will hurt for a couple of hours and then go again.' Believe me, it's wonderful for the ego to be told the next week how brilliant you are because it happened exactly as you said it would. But of course none of this is new. It is 2000 years since Jesus said, 'It is your own faith which has cured you.'

Using suggestibility to improve a person's attitude towards their own health is usually the domain of the hypnotherapist. Though most hypnotherapists tend to treat emotional problems, an increasing number of them are also getting involved in physical healing.

What about doctors in all this? They have a great responsibility, not only for the treatment they prescribe but also for the words they use. Quite often the words they use will more effectively kill or cure than the disease or treatment can. When someone is told in the consultant's private office, that they have been diagnosed as having cancer, or multiple sclerosis, or some other terrible ailment, they immediately go into a state of shock.

They are often, unintentionally, made to feel insignificant, inferior or overawed by a white-coated surgeon or consultant and talked to in a langauge which they can barely hear and are less likely to understand. The shock becomes so overwhelming that they can only pick up key words, such as 'cancer', 'serious', 'three months'. In a situation like this the patient is reduced to a hypnotic state, which means that the logical consciousness is bypassed and the key words go directly into the subconscious. The logical consciousness is knocked out by the stress which has been induced through fear and shock. It then becomes impossible to reason logically and, as the intellect switches off, the key words go directly to that area of the brain responsible for obeying the instructions fed into it, the subconscious.

The consultant is unwittingly programming his patient's computer to self-destruct. By making predictions to someone in a hypnotic state of shock, he will cause his own predictions to come true. Having now primed the time bomb with a sequence of commands, and leaving no instructions on how to switch it off, he embarks on a series of treatments which are rarely successful, always horrendous, painful and dehumanising.

The words doctors use in these situations can kill or cure, cause fear or calm. I will not dwell on this point though it is something I feel passionately about. I will simply illustrate what I mean with a classic example.

A woman phoned to make an appointment in the hope that I could cure her frozen shoulder. These can sometimes be freed in minutes and sometimes, especially if it's been going on a long time, it can take several visits. This particular case was one of the easier ones. In about five minutes her shoulder was free.

As she had booked for a half-hour session I asked her if she had any other problems. Then I noticed that her left arm was strangely limp, though it was the right shoulder I had just treated. She explained that about three years earlier she had had a mild stroke and it had left her with a paralysed arm. At the time she had had other problems but these had more or less corrected themselves and it was just the arm which remained lifeless.

I took the affected arm in my hand and thought that it felt surprisingly light for a paralysed arm. In a normal arm there is an electrical current and around the arm an electromagnetic field which counteracts gravitational pull. After a stroke, when the nerves have been damaged and the flow of electricity to an area prevented, that area usually loses its electromagnetic field and feels very heavy. The lightness in this case indicated to me that the nerve functions were all in order and I could find no reason why the arm should not work.

So I gently lifted her useless arm until it was straight up in the air, my own electromagnetic field reinforcing hers. I told her to hold it there, above her head. I then went and sat on a low stool, which I placed directly in front of her, looked her straight in the eyes and said, 'Lower your arm,' which she did.

Still holding her gaze I instructed her to raise her paralysed arm above her head, which she did. At this point I just grinned. A look of disbelief crossed her face and then she got up and went dancing around the room, waving her arm in the air, proclaiming that God had worked a miracle through me, that I was truly a spiritual healer. At this point I began to worry. I could see hundreds of stroke sufferers coming to my door expecting miracle cures, like some poor man's Lourdes, so I did some fast explaining.

At the time of her stroke she would have been in a state of shock, unable to reason, taking in literally everything that was said to her by the white-coated man in authority. This kindly gentleman had casually told her, 'You probably won't be able to use that arm again.' Being in a hypnotic state of shock her subconscious had picked that sentence up as an instruction. And so, even when the shock and symptoms of stroke had long passed the subconscious doggedly stuck to the instruction that the arm was useless. It was only when someone of greater authority or mental power came along to countermand that instruction that she could take control of her arm once more. This is by no means an isolated case; I have had many.

Of course, if there had been any physical damage to the brain as a result of the stroke I could not have cured it. Where there is permanent damage I cannot alter the situation and it is blatantly false for any healer to claim miracle cures for himself or God when no such thing has occurred. I am sure that every single case of a cure through a visit to Lourdes is a direct result of the holy water's reputation being mightier than the situation which caused the paralysis. Those who go to Lourdes are cured by their faith, which breaks the hypnotic belief or suggestion implanted in their minds when they were in a state of shock. Similar cures can be seen in some church services when the congregation is worked up into a state of hypnotic fervour and various emotional or shock-induced infirmities are cured.

At the risk of being excommunicated, stoned to death, burnt at the stake, or whatever it is they do these days to anyone who questions such beliefs, I can state categorically that God does not choose to heal one person while leaving another untreated because of some difference in religious belief. I have had situations where people have literally 'picked up their bed and walked', but my only claim is that I see and feel the inner need of these people for love and understanding. It is this and nothing more which gives me the ability to help others.

Trauma can be released in any situation which raises emotions to the hysteria state. Typical situations are religious or evangelical meetings. They can be the size of those held in Wembley Stadium. Or they can be small groups which, either through prayers or music, create a hypnotic or hysteria state which will cause a trauma release in certain types of individuals. At the point of trauma release the subconscious allows the logical mind full responsibility for the physical state once again, thus curing psychosomatic conditions. However, there are two dangers in this. The first is that the trauma may only be partially released, leaving the person concerned in a state of emotional instability. The second danger is that the congregation, having been worked up into a condition of high emotion, enters a hypnotic state. As such, it is very vulnerable to suggestion by the minister in charge of the service. These are perfect conditions for brain-washing. Hitler was a master of the art.

Perfectly innocent ministers and religious leaders, and some less innocent, do untold damage to susceptible and immature congregations, especially with talk of judgement and other fear-based statements. Fear-induced illness is probably the biggest single factor affecting health, and anything or anyone who creates fear in the mind of another for whatever reason is guilty of adversely affecting that person's health.

PHOBIAS

I make no distinction between phobia, depression and emotional stress or allergies. They all have the same origin, unreleased fear resulting in repressed emotion which, one way or another, continues to haunt its victim until it is released.

Anne's particular phobia was a fear of feathers which, for those interested in long names, is called pteronophobia. I stood behind Anne and asked her to relax for a minute or two. Then, when I felt I had reduced her brain-wave frequency to the change-state level, I asked her to recall the first time she had felt this fear of feathers. Her subconscious was only too pleased to release the thoughts of fear which had been causing the negative emotions. She began to remember quite distinctly being taken as a child of three into a building full of turkeys which were being killed for Christmas. She described the scene in graphic detail from a little girl's viewpoint. Feathers up to her knees, feathers floating around her face, a feeling of suffocating in feathers. Anne was terrified that the turkeys which were still running loose and seemingly twice her size, would attack her. She had to watch them struggling in fear and panic as they were chased, caught and killed in a quite barbaric way, and then feathers, feathers and more feathers. People were laughing at her as she stood petrified and screaming and then she remembered being told off for being silly. Eventually she was lifted up and taken outside.

The subconscious had no difficulty in repressing that memory, but whenever it was confronted with anything representing a feather it sent out warning signals of panic and fear. Now that this childhood trauma had been brought to the surface Anne the woman could take over from Anne the child. The memory was brought into proper perspective and caused no more problems. Once the cause of a phobia has been recalled and released it ceases to be.

Agoraphobia

Another phobia which I think is fairly common is agoraphobia — a fear of open spaces. This particular client, Alice, had had no signs of her phobia until, in her mid-forties, she suddenly found herself beginning to panic every time she left home or walked out of shops into the street. It all began about six months after her father died and it was generally considered that it was the shock of losing her father which had brought it on. The situation persisted for many years before Alice eventually found her way to my front door. By this time she had had the usual counselling, drugs and therapy, all to no avail. As she said, the phobia had completely destroyed her enjoyment of life. The point had been reached where she didn't go out anywhere. Her friends no longer called and it was badly affecting her marriage.

The big difficulty with emotional problems is that they can't be seen. So, unless your friends have experienced it for themselves, there isn't likely to be much sympathy. The usual advice is 'Pull yourself together', 'stop being silly', but this doesn't work because it's our old friend the subconscious taking control of things again. The subconscious has been conditioned by past experience and is immune to logical reasoning. I put my hands over Alice's head and caused her to go into the changed-state of consciousness. It only took about five minutes and she was soon able to remember the first time she had felt panic in the streets. She had been about four, her father had taken her to the local town for a day's shopping. Somehow she wandered from her father's side and out on to the street. Try to imagine, if you can, how it must feel to be a four-year-old. The pavement, the shops, the cars all seem several times bigger than they are now. A little girl suddenly realising that she is on her own, lost, in a big wide street, being towered over by unsmiling, unknown people who are all rushing about, feels very insecure. You feel so small and the people around you look like giants. All you can see are legs. There is no sense of distance because you can't see over people.

It was interesting that the first thought which went through Alice's mind was not 'Where is Daddy?' but 'How will I get my food, where will I sleep, who will put me to bed?' I've noticed before that people who can clearly recall childhood trauma rarely think of their parents first, their thoughts nearly always go to survival. By the time Alice's father found her she had worked herself up into a right old panic. Her fear about how she would cope was intense. Of course as soon as her father found her the panic subsided, she got the usual telling-off and was told, 'if you lose me again stay inside by the door.' It was then all forgotten. But not by our ever-watchful friend, the subconscious. This ever-alert controller who is responsible for our survival forgets nothing. And when Alice's father died forty years later the subconscious recalled vividly what happened last time she was separated from her father. That time, when she was four, Alice panicked and the subconscious took instructions from that incident which it carefully noted. The instructions were, if I lose my father I must stay inside or I panic.

The subconscious is quite unconcerned about details such as age difference. It has its instructions. 'If I get separated from father, stay inside'. When Alice's father died and someone said to her, 'I'm sorry you've lost your father,' her subconscious created a panic right on cue, and it continued to do all it could to prevent Alice from going into open spaces until her father could be found. Once again, when the adult Alice remembered and understood the incident, the subconscious gave up responsibility for the situation and her phobia quickly dissolved.

So much for helping other people overcome their phobias. What happens when the healer himself has a phobia? People seem to assume that being a healer automatically ensures that I am never ill, or that if I am I can quickly overcome the problem by giving myself healing. Unfortunately it isn't quite that simple. I wish it were. If my legs hurt or I twist something or I get backache it's very difficult to put my own hands on the troubled area. And anyway I can't affect my own energy level with my own energy level, so physical healing as described in the earlier parts of this book isn't really practical. I therefore use self-hypnosis to heal myself.

I know this sounds difficult but it's only a form of meditation. What I do is to leave my body in a spiritual sense and see myself from a distance (more about this in Part III). Then I am quite capable of sending healing energies into my 'distant' body. It's very effective. The trick, of course, is being able to see yourself from somewhere else and the best time to do this is just as you are dropping off to sleep. If you can, just as you begin to slip towards sleep, feel your body becoming heavier but let your spirit remain awake. Once you have achieved this, you will have effectively put yourself into deep self-hypnosis, and in that state anything is possible. If you have a problem, physical or emotional, this self-hypnotic state will allow you to examine it. This time I'll use a situation I found myself in as an example.

As far as I know I'm not afraid of anything, certainly not dying. It has always been my view that what becomes of my body, once I've lost interest in it, isn't really my problem. Burial or cremation, it really doesn't matter, I won't be there and provided someone clears away the bits and pieces I leave behind I'm just not bothered. But all that began to change in the early spring of 1992. I didn't know why but I began to think that perhaps being cremated was not such a good idea.

At first I didn't even realise that my views had changed. It was so gradual, so subtle, but very definite. The more I thought about it, the more I began to reject the idea of cremation. At this point it hadn't even crossed my mind to wonder why I should be thinking about it anyway. As the weeks passed the idea of being cremated began to seem more and more repulsive. Eventually I decided to write to the Nottingham School of Medicine offering my body for research. Anything, I thought, would be better than being cremated. I sat down and wrote quite a good letter really, in view of the fact that I was offering my body for research at least forty years before they could expect to take delivery!

At this point I suddenly came to my senses. These were the symptoms of a phobia, so the first question to ask was, what triggered the fear? For the first time I sat down and thought it through in detail. I had been feeling like this for about three months, so, what happened about three to four months ago? It must have been something to do with cremation or burning. I hadn't been to any funerals, I didn't know anyone who had been burnt, ah — wait a minute. My daughter-in-law had burnt her hands on the grill about then. She had burnt the palms of her hands and had had to have them treated in hospital. It wasn't serious, but she had needed treatment and her hands had been bandaged. So that's why the subconscious sent me a warning. But why?

There was only one thing for it. I had to get myself to go back through my life. So, using the self induced hypnotic state described earlier, I started to journey back through my memories. I knew that it had to be a childhood trauma of some kind and because I was tuned in to it, it didn't take many minutes to find the cause of my fear of cremation.

When I was about four or five I slipped in front of an open coal fire and fell into it. Naturally I put my hands out to prevent the fall and little hands burn very easily. My mother was there and yanked me out quickly, but not before I had badly burnt the palms of my hands. It was a very frightening experience. In my hypnotic state I relived the whole episode and the thought going through my panicking mind as I fell and before I hit the fire was, 'I don't want to burn'.

Now I had the connection. When I heard about my daughter-in-law burning the palms of her hands my subconscious sent up the panic warning, 'I don't want to burn.' But it forgot to tell me that it related to falling into the fire when I was little. I therefore interpreted the message according to my current age and somehow that got twisted to cremation. If I hadn't been able to trace my own emotions through logic and memory release I would most probably have gone through the rest of my life feeling terrified in case I was cremated. As it is, I'm afraid the world of medical science has lost a most interesting collection of antique bones.

Allergies

I have noticed that many allergies are a form of phobia. I have had several clients whose allergic reaction to sugar or milk was the direct result of a childhood trauma which for some reason they had cause to react to later in life.

One client I recall asked if I could do anything about an

allergy he had to milk. He had first noticed a problem seven years earlier and the allergy had become so extreme that he was unable to consume any food which contained milk. As many of the foods we eat include milk products in one way or another his life had become very difficult. He told me that the allergy had first been noticed soon after his wife left him. Using the usual healing techniques he was able to recall his early childhood and remembered that his mother had left his father when he was just a few months old because his father had become an alcoholic. He was 'hitting the bottle' as he put it. The connection was easy to make. The child's subconscious had noted that drinking too much from the bottle caused father to lose his wife. Of course at that age he assumed it was milk in the bottle which father drank. Now move on forty years. His wife leaves him, he wants her back, subconscious recalls the early memory and so starts rejecting all milk products. A subconscious desire to save the marriage. Of course at a logical level this is never understood but once the connection is made the allergy starts to subside. The subconscious has got its message across. This is not a unique case. I have had several very similar cases.

Alcoholism

Another condition which I have come to realise is sometimes phobic in origin is alcoholism. Normally I won't see alcoholics because they need specialist treatment which I am not trained to give. One particular woman, however, phoned to ask if I would help her with her drink problem. Something about her story just didn't fit with the problems normally associated with alcoholics, so I agreed to see her and she duly arrived one Friday evening.

Her story was that she had started to drink, or 'hit the bottle' as she preferred to call it, soon after her baby was born. She noticed that she was beginning to resent the family or friends calling in to see either her or the baby, and it reached ridiculous proportions when she even tried to prevent her own husband from seeing their baby. She would scheme, there is no other word for it, to ensure that the child was in bed before the father came home from work and not roused until after he had left again early in the morning.

Of course she wasn't always successful. Her husband would insist on going to see his baby and there was nothing she could do about his being with the baby at weekends. It was then that she noticed that whenever anyone else, including her husband, spent time with her baby she would have to have a drink. As the baby got older and she was less able to prevent family, friends or neighbours from seeing or playing with her baby, so her drink problem intensified.

'It was no good,' she said. 'It got that whenever anyone visited the house I would hit the bottle, especially after they had gone.'

When she came to see me she was truly alcoholic, or was she? When we delved deep into her childhood history it became apparent that her mother had often forgotten to give her her bottle-feed, especially if someone had called around for a chat. In fact this happened on so many occasions that she began to resent people calling at the house. As a baby she quickly associated people calling at the house with a missed bottle-feed. Twenty-three years later she had a baby of her own. And her subconscious said, 'I remember being a baby. It means if people call around I don't get my bottle.'

Unfortunately the subconscious is unable to make any allowance for age difference or type of bottle. Once the phobia is set in motion with the arrival of the baby and its association with memories of her own baby years, the victim, now a grown adult, is caused to crave for a bottle every time someone calls at her home. But a drink from a bottle to an adult, who can't translate subconscious cravings, means alcohol. Once the cause of the problem was understood, it could be dealt with.

EMOTIONS

Emotions are built-in reactions to current or past situations. Virtually every emotion we experience is a programmed response. That program was formulated when we were very young and one of the most health-damaging emotions that can be taught is fear. Fear is all right if it allows us to escape a life-threatening situation or reminds us to avoid a dangerous situation, such as eating wild berries when we are young or playing in the traffic. But when we are taught to unconsciously react in fear to another's opinion of us then we have entered a rogue reaction into our subconscious.

The biggest problem with fear is that it prevents us from doing things. It's like a brake which prevents us experiencing new situations and the hand on the brake is usually someone else's. How many of you reading this book, I wonder, would like to do something different in your life, today, but resist doing anything about it simply because of what someone else might say. This is fear. Fear of the opinions others may have about you. Fear of disapproval.

A lot of my time is spent as a counsellor, helping people overcome problems which prevent them from enjoying life to the full. In fact I would go further than that and say that many of the people who come to me with stress or emotional depression are in that state simply because they fear the negative opinions which others may have about them.

The moment your partner, friend or associate and especially your enemy realise that you need their approval in some area of life, you are doomed to become a slave to their moral blackmail.

Disapproval is something we learn about in our early years. I'm sure you remember phrases like, 'Don't do that or Daddy will be cross', 'Don't do that or it will upset Mummy', 'Don't do that, it makes the teacher angry', 'Don't do that, what would the doctor say,' and hundreds of other similar sentences, all designed to program your emotions so that you never do anything which anyone might disapprove of. Without realising it you have been programmed into 'inaction' because someone, somewhere, is bound to disapprove, whatever you do.

But surely that is their problem, not yours. If somebody doesn't like what you are doing or saying, and provided that what you are doing is not harming their interests, then surely the way they feel about it is of no importance. To bring you back into line, just in case you do decide to kick the fear habit, you will be told that you are selfish for not considering others. I maintain that the selfish person is the one who is using the emotional blackmail because that is what it most certainly is.

This became apparent to me very early on in my life. I had been out with a couple of friends. I suppose we were about seven years old at the time. It was a wet, muddy sort of a day, and after having a good tramp around in the fields and with mud up to our knees, we decided to go into one of my friend's homes for a drink. Of course, we didn't think to take our muddy Wellingtons off. Straight into the kitchen we went, our boots leaving a lovely, dirty trail across the kitchen floor. Understandably, the lady of the house was not amused.

'Get out of here you dirty little tykes,' she yelled, or something like that. We didn't hang around long enough to offer any explanations. Her body langauge was already indicating that flight was our best course of action. Her parting shot was, 'Kids, they make me sick.'

At that age our survival skills were not too well developed and so we did the same thing again at my other friend's home. This time, however, the reaction was totally different. The three of us, complete with muddy Wellingtons, trudged across the nice clean kitchen floor but instead of screaming abuse at us and saying we made her feel sick, his mother started to laugh, and told us to get up on to a stool while she got us a drink and biscuits. She then took our Wellingtons off and with a smile said, 'O.K. boys, the bucket is in the corner, the cloth is under the sink. It's your mud, put it back outside.'

At that point I learned a big lesson. We hadn't made the first mother angry or sick; she had chosen to be angry and feel sick. This mother had chosen to be amused and laugh. I had come to realise that we choose our emotions. Nobody makes us angry, envious, jealous, sad or happy. We choose for ourselves how we feel, we choose which emotion is best for us. The trouble is that most of us have been emotionally programmed when we were small always to try and anticipate how others will react and avoid any action which might cause them to react negatively. Some people take this conditioning to such lengths that they spend their whole lives worrying about what others will think or do. They worry about responses over which they have no control. This is fear; it is a brake on normal creative activities.

And what of your own emotions? I have had people tell me that they have been insulted by a friend. No they haven't. They have chosen to feel insulted. We choose our emotions; nobody chooses them for us. Positive emotions help us to avoid health- damaging thoughts. Probably the biggest factor in the survival game is being able to avoid negative emotions. Let's examine a few.

Fear

I've already said this is probably the most health-damaging of all the emotions. In most people it is there all the time. People dress so as not to cause offence and are then fearful that they might not have succeeded and later spend time worrying because someone said something which they interpreted, possibly wrongly, to mean what they did was not acceptable. There is no way out of this trap except to reprogramme your computer to respond with positive thoughts. If you don't, sooner or later fear will cause a breakdown somewhere in your system.

Anger

This is an emotion we choose as an antidote to fear. In trying to come to terms with the emotion of fear we blame others. As

Dr Wayne Dyer put it in his book *Your Erroneous Zones*, 'The only antidote to anger is to eliminate the internal sentence "If only you were more like me."' Having programmed ourselves to be fearful, we then try to override the program with one of anger. We try to blame the other person because we feel fear or guilt or some other negative emotion. But using a second negative to cancel the first is no answer at all.

We need to remember the basic point that it doesn't matter what other people do or think. If you are going to be angry don't blame anyone else. You chose the anger when you could have chosen to ignore the incident or at least been unemotional about it. Anger releases bioelectricity in huge quantities. And why should other people think like you, or do as you suppose they should? Harbouring anger or its more aggressive brother, hate, in your heart is sure to cause you immense pain.

Maybe somebody you know has caused a difficulty in your life, but is your anger going to alter what has happened? I doubt it. And how do you think the other person will respond to your anger? They will respond in the same way you did by being angry and expecting you to be like them. And so it goes on, each one expecting the other to change so that they can avoid the emotion of fear. All these negative emotions cause disease and ill health, a breakdown in the normal scheme of things.

Jealousy

Jealousy is an emotion which is also based on fear, a fear of loss. To try and eliminate that fear we put conditions on the giving of love. It is love which the jealous are frightened of losing, or not receiving. Jealousy is a basic inadequacy, fear of losing something which in their hearts they know they don't own anyway. So, to overcome their fear of loss they use fear as a weapon. 'I'll love you on condition that ...' If you take away all the conditions from your love, jealousy no longer has any basis.

Love should always be unconditional. If it isn't then it's not love. You don't love someone if you add the words, or thoughts, 'on condition that ...'. Jealousy is a terrible emotion which eats away at the soul. It poisons the body as it poisons thoughts and those who choose this emotion choose ill-health. Better to be rid of your passion than be consumed with jealousy which eats away at you until your features become a reflection of your contorted thoughts and fears.

Guilt and Worry

Guilt and worry are two emotions which often go together. This is because people who feel guilty about a past thought or action worry about it into the future. Again both these emotions are based on fear, fear about what has been done and what others will think or do about what you have done. What a total waste of time this is.

'It's easy to say that,' I can hear you thinking, 'but I can't help worrying about what I've done, or am going to do.' Why can't you stop yourself worrying? Quite simply because your subconscious, your auto-pilot, your computer, was programmed in your early years to know fear so that others could call you civilised. Now I am not against morality or a civilised way of behaving based on self-discipline. But that self-discipline should be based on love of others, not fear of others. There is no negative emotion that is not based on fear and every one of them is a self-destruct device. You were programmed to respect fear at an early age as a means of keeping you under control. If you let go of fear you can begin to think independently.

Every week I see clients who are destroying themselves with negative emotions, such as jealousy, guilt, envy, anger or, to sum them up in one word, fear. Think of all the cases I've cited so far which are subconsciously caused; they are all based on fear in one form or another. The problem is that this fear is passed from one generation to the next. As you were taught, so you teach. I get many clients who are deeply distressed and suffering from arthritis, stomach problems, heart or respiratory trouble and who, in general conversation while I'm healing them, tell me that it's their children, or parents, or friends who have caused them to feel down and depressed: 'And after all we've done for them.' A nice little bit of moral blackmail that.

Whatever emotion these people feel, it's because they have chosen it, because they wanted to control the emotions of their children or friends. They could have chosen love and happiness but they didn't. And however much they blame others there's no getting away from the fact that the way they feel is the way they have chosen to feel, and the way they think is reflected in their overall health. We are all a reflection of what we think. Fear, in all its forms, is destructive. There is only one constructive and healthy emotion, love. This gives birth to all the positive emotions of joy, compassion and happiness.

Whatever emotions you feel don't ever blame another; you chose them. Your thoughts are your power. They can build your life or they can destroy it. As you choose your thoughts, so you choose your health. As the Buddha said, 'The mind is everything; what you think you become.'

ARTHRITIS

I had quite a lot of difficulty deciding in which part of the book to include this particular health problem. Some types of arthritis, such as rheumatoid can be made much worse by emotional stress, while osteo-arthritis is more likely to be caused by a physical injury. However it didn't seem right to divide the subject of arthritis between different parts of the book so I've opted to include all arthritis in this one section.

There are many different types of arthritis. I remember reading somewhere that over forty different types have been identified, but for me they fall into three main categories: rheumatoid, osteo and rheumatism.

Rheumatoid Arthritis

Of the three, rheumatoid arthritis must rank as the worst. It really is a crippling disease which is not at all selective about which area of the body it chooses to show itself in. On one day it might be pain in the elbows and the next day perhaps the knees.

Personally I can't say that healing is wonderfully effective when the symptoms are at their worst, unless it is treated as psychosomatic. Otherwise relief is usually short-lived and the patient needs to return at least once a week, sometimes for several weeks, or even months, to retain any advantages that the healing may have given. This is not to say that another healer would not do better and I am sure there are healers around the country who have an excellent record of treating and perhaps curing rheumatoid arthritis without getting involved in deeper emotional causes.

However, once the worst of the condition has passed, healing can have a dramatic effect. The problem is knowing if the condition is in temporary remission or has actually burnt itself out. I know one woman whose rheumatoid arthritis was just as active and crippling in her eighties as it had been twenty years earlier. I also know a woman who at thirty-two seemed to have beaten the disease. She had first been diagnosed as having rheumatoid arthritis when she was seventeen. Shock was the cause. She became pregnant at sixteen, and twelve months later was in a terrible state. By the time she was thirty she was a virtual cripple with stiff joints and almost unusable limbs. But at thirty-two she had recovered from the shock of sixteen years earlier and there was no sign of the pain or other symptoms except of course for the long-term damage caused to her joints. It was at this point that I was asked to help.

Week after week, month after month, this lady returned for healing until after about twelve months she could again walk unaided, climb stairs and use her fingers, hands and arms. She would always have the tell-tale signs of this awful complaint but she was pain-free, independent and mobile.

Another case I remember was of a young girl whose wrist, elbow and shoulder joints were very severely affected, though she could go for long periods without any pain or swellings. It was during one of those better periods that she came for help. Almost immediately her stiffened joints began to improve, the pain receded and some freedom returned. Then, after a few weeks, she came on a routine visit and her joints were hot, swollen and very, very painful. For some reason the condition had returned, with a vengeance.

It has been my experience that sometimes this problem is caused, or made worse, by extreme emotions such as jealousy, anger or fear, and when the emotions subside so do the symptoms. I questioned the young lady and eventually she reluctantly told me that she had had a blazing argument with her boyfriend who had then walked out on her. This is just the sort of situation which will bring on an attack. When she calmed down, so did the painful symptoms.

At a later date we decided to find the original cause of her condition and in a hypnotic state she released the emotions of a sexual attack which had taken place when she was a teenager. Held down by her arms during the attack, she had struggled violently to free herself. After that any emotion or argument involving the opposite sex brought on the symptoms of pain and swelling in her hands and arms. This was a subconscious reaction to an emotional threat, though she had no recall of the ordeal because her subconscious had repressed the memory of it. Neither had she ever told anyone of the attack. After releasing the repressed emotions in the healing session I don't think she has suffered another attack of rheumatoid arthritis and this was several years ago.

Rheumatoid arthritis is very much an emotional condition, though this may not always be easy to see. Healers are probably most effective when they are capable of releasing or identifying the emotion which is causing or has caused the symptoms to appear.

Only recently a lady came to me who had suffered from

rheumatoid arthritis for ten years. She told me that she was affected mostly in her knees, wrists and the top of her spine. I asked her what had happened during the year immediately before the arthritis first became apparent. She went quiet for a minute or two before telling me of the death of two close friends. But there was more. This was apparent because of the silence which followed, so I waited.

Then she told me about another friend who had committed suicide, because of loneliness, on a day when she was in the area where the friend was living. This had left her with a great feeling of guilt.

I then asked her if she was religious. She replied, 'No, but as a child I was brought up as a Catholic. But I no longer go to church though I still have my faith.'

'When you were little and had done something wrong what did you do?' I asked.

There was a long pause, 'I went and said a prayer to Jesus.'

'How did you do that?'

'I knelt beside the bed on my knees, with my hands together and my head bowed.'

'Now do you see why you have your pains? Your subconscious is telling you that to purge your guilt you must say a prayer — hence the pain in your knees, your wrists and the top of your spine.'

A week later she told me that all her guilt had left her and her pain was also practically gone.

Because healing brings peace of mind and contentment it can have a very beneficial effect on emotional problems of all types, though until the cause is identified and dealt with the condition is always likely to return.

Osteo-Arthritis

Osteo-arthritis is usually caused by injury or damage to the joints and most of the cases I see are the results of sporting injuries. These I find particularly satisfying to treat, in that there is usually a high success rate. While I am putting my hands over the afflicted areas there are often the most disgusting cracking and creaking noises as the solidified joints begin to respond. But the treatment is quite painless, despite the gruesome sounds. It really is like watching a miracle as previously immovable joints loosen and begin to move at the first healing session.

I remember one particular man who had contracted his osteo-arthritis as a professional footballer. Now in his sixties he had to limp his way around the golf course, but after just one session he was able to enjoy a comfortable round of golf. This was exceptional of course, and he had to come many more times before the improvement was permanent. Even so, I could give many examples of successfully treated osteo-arthritis. For sheer ego-boosting, I suppose this ailment is a healer's dream.

This is a condition which should rightly have gone into the first section of the book because it is one's own bioelectricity stimulating another's muscle movements which causes the extraordinary results. I know that many healers will consider this statement sacrilegious because they believe that all healing comes from God and that healers are only a channel. Well, I'm not going to get involved in any arguments about it but the energy which causes an osteo-arthritis cure is physical and not metaphysical. And I'm sure that low-frequency pulsed electricity would have exactly the same effect.

Rheumatism

Rheumatism is what most people, including me, call any condition where the joints swell, particularly in the hands, causing a lot of pain. Unfortunately most people don't go for treatment until it is too late and then blame the doctor for not being able to do anything about it. If people with painful joints go to a healer, and they are now in plentiful supply all over the country, they should be able to get the relief they are looking for. I don't particularly believe that drugs are the answer, and they often seem to cause as many problems as they cure.

Worn hips, I think, come under this heading. Like other joints, hips become worn because the muscles supporting and moving them often become too tight, pulling the bones on to one another. The joint then wears, causing awful pain. Healing will not make a worn hip whole again. But it will relax the muscles around the joint, freeing it to work normally. And if the joint can be freed then very often all the pain disappears.

I had one case where the person concerned was due to go for a hip replacement operation in six to eight weeks time but because the pain was so unbearable she came to see if I could do anything to relieve it in the meantime. She came with a friend who helped her into the treatment room and she used a stick for extra support. Her hip had totally seized up, making it very painful and difficult to get around.

In these sort of situations I hold the patient's ankle and let my energy flow up through the leg. In just a few minutes her whole leg began to tremble, then shake and jump as, one by one, the muscles began to relax. At the end of the half-hour session she could walk almost perfectly and the pain had gone. She went back to her doctor, who sent her for another examination which confirmed that the joint was now free. Not that confirmation was necessary, of course. The improvement in mobility and freedom from pain were entirely due to relaxing the muscles so that the joint was free again. She decided not to go ahead with the operation and, three years later, she is still pain free and mobile.

Incidentally I've also been asked to treat frozen hip joints which I have not been able to help. This is not a negative approach, but I don't want people who read this to think that all hip joint problems can be cured by healing because it isn't so. What I am saying is that in all but the very severe cases I can relieve the joints and sometimes an operation becomes unnecessary, especially if the problem is brought to me very early.

PART III

THE EJECTOR SEAT

Spiritual Healing

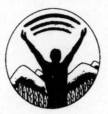

P arts I and II of this book have been about life-giving physical energy and the emotional energy which influences its character. It is through this combination of energies that we are able to experience life. Both physical and emotional energy are part of the life experience but when we die, and move to other dimensions, we have no need of them. At this point we become spirit energy once again. Spiritual energy is the essence of awareness; it is who we are. Vegetable matter radiates energy in a way similar to that of our bodies but it lacks the emotion which would allow it to change its inherent structure. Animals are the same as ourselves except their ability to experience emotion is limited to the capacity of their mind or reasoning powers. They are also spirit but lower emotional capacity limits their use of expression and awareness. Spiritual energy is awareness expressed as love and it is this energy or awareness, which is separate from the body, that we now move on to discuss.

Leaving the body is very much like pressing the ejector seat button in a plane which is falling apart and can no longer hold you.

In this final section we examine how the pilot communicates and experiences life without the protection of his plane. We explain the difference between permanent and temporary separation from the plane which has been our world. We go on to put the case for reincarnation and how previous lives can affect our health in this life.

Pressing the Button

I estimate that possibly up to 20 per cent of the population have an extra perception which the other 80 per cent lack. This is because the spirit, or consciousness, has not become totally one with its physical body. It has therefore retained its spiritual perception and is able to use it independently, in addition to physical perception. This allows the spirit to provide the brain with information which would not normally be available to it. And these extra sensations are of a frequency which is beyond the that of the physical.

SHIFT IN CONSCIOUSNESS

As I explained at the beginning of this book, when the foetus begins to develop, a spirit joins with it. However until birth the spirit is not totally one with the physical body it is joining. And even after birth it takes many years before the spirit is so totally enmeshed with the physical body that it loses its spiritual awareness. The exact number of years that it takes spirit and body to become one varies from child to child but, as a general rule, a spirit is not totally one with the body it is using until about its seventh year. This is why so many young children talk about playing with supposedly non-existent people. These people do exist, but not to an adult who has lost the separate perception of the spirit and has to rely totally on physical senses.

During old age, assuming that we are maturing normally, the spirit begins to disengage from the web of the physical, so the elderly begin once again to perceive with their spirit as well as their physical bodies. This is why it is usually those above middle-age who report psychic phenomena and why those who have passed middle-age are more able to accept spiritualism and the revelations of a greater dimension. Maturing and young to middle-aged adults tend to be without spirit perceptions.

Of course there are always exceptions and these are the 20 per cent I speak of. The deeper spiritual perception of this 20 per cent ranges from very slight to total. It is this extra perception, beyond that of the physical, which is known as clairvoyance, clairaudience and so on. It means learning to perceive with spirit awareness instead of mind and body consciousness and this is what I refer to as a shift in consciousness.

Those who have retained some measure of spiritual independence find it virtually impossible to explain this extra depth of perception to those who lack it. Having extra perception allows one to experience a wider dimension. (A dimension is no more than a band of electromagnetic frequencies that the human body can perceive or recognise.) The spirit, which vibrates at a much higher frequency than the physical, can sense or perceive electromagnetic frequencies which are beyond the limits of the physical. As we have seen, by the time it is in its seventh year, the spirit has normally become so enmeshed with the body it is using that it is unable to recognise the higher frequencies which were once available to it. For those with spirit perception or awareness, the meaning of reality is totally different. Sometimes, of course, individuals who are totally locked into the physical will experience psychic phenomena brought on by stress. Occasionally this happens as flashes of insight or intuition. It is these differences in awareness between people, and in the same people at different times, that have given rise to a belief in different levels of consciousness. In fact there is only one consciousness and it is complete in itself; it does not have different levels. Absolute consciousness is spiritual awareness. Other levels of consciousness such as the subconscious are the archives of the mind. They are part of physical awareness and should not be confused with spiritual awareness.

SPIRITUAL HEALING

Many of us begin to think about spiritual matters when we lose someone who is dear to us. I mentioned earlier the physical aspect of grieving which is akin to depression. In no way should this be compared to the spiritual aspect of grieving which is on a totally different plane. While your partner was alive in the flesh it was easy to use the physical senses to communicate love, but when that method is withdrawn it becomes necessary to move to higher levels of awareness and cause yourself to be aware of spiritual love. If you look for and experience spiritual love and spiritual awareness you will find again that love which you had thought had gone forever.

Many, many people come to me suffering from the grief of loss. They are usually able to experience the presence of the love they had thought was gone because, through the healing experience, they are able to lift themselves into a new world of spiritual awareness. And this, in case you are thinking it, has nothing to do with spiritualism. Healing love causes a shift in consciousness by first taking the client from physical perception into emotional perception and then as the healing intensifies it moves away from the emotional block of the subconscious and into true spiritual awareness. All earthly problems and bodily ailments are then seen with true spiritual perception and dismissed for what they are, passing experiences.

This is spiritual healing which needs no explanation. This

level of healing is not acquired with training or logic, but those who are capable of radiating such totally unselfish love are few in number. There can be no explanation for its success because spiritual love does not seek success or gain; it just is. Such people radiate love wherever they go. They are not necessarily the famous or the worldly, though they might be; they can just as easily be unknown, except by those around them who are drawn to their peace and contentment.

Why, I hear you asking, have I gone to such lengths to describe physical healing, involving psychology and electro-magnetic fields, in the earlier part of this book, if spiritual healing can so easily bypass the physical and emotional elements to free the individual of trauma and pain? The reason is that not everyone is ready for a shift in consciousness. Many do not believe, or their own spiritual love is not readily available to help them see beyond physical perception and its false reality. For these people the body and mind still need to be understood by the body and mind, and healing needs to be logically explained and administered. But usually, once the miracle of spiritual healing has been experienced, even unwittingly, the shift in consciousness will begin. Depth of awareness and purpose will increase as the spirit becomes responsible for expression and the emotions of fear are brought under control.

I think I can best illustrate this particular point by referring to a young lady who came to me with infertility problems. As I explained earlier in the book many cases of infertility are caused by nothing more than stress, which is utilisation of energy in greater quantities than are readily available. When the body doesn't have the resources to sustain a growing foetus without causing problems for the mother it uses subconscious control to prevent a pregnancy or reject the foetus immediately after conception. However there are often spiritual reasons why a woman will not fall pregnant. In the following case it was a mixture of subconscious rejection and spiritual insecurity which was preventing a pregnancy.

The young lady was slightly built and, though nervous about

coming to see me, seemed very sure of herself. She had a responsible and demanding full-time job. Her husband, whom I was to meet later, had a secure job and was an easy-going, undemanding character. Both of them desperately wanted children, but after being married for eight years and being told by doctors that there was no obvious reason why they should not have started a family they both began to doubt that they ever would.

At our first meeting I went into the usual explanation of the need to keep energy levels up, though it was already obvious that the reason for the woman's infertility was something other than nutritional. She came every week for several weeks, during which time she began to undergo a change in consciousness. Eventually we reached the point where I could help her to perceive spiritually the cause of her infertility.

I asked her to close her eyes and see a blackboard. When she could confirm that the blackboard was visible to her imagination I asked her to draw a big white circle on it. Again, before moving on, I asked her to confirm that she had been able to do this. From this point on I only moved to the next step after she confirmed that she had been able to do the action I had just talked her through. When she had drawn her circle I asked her to take a cloth and wipe out the board inside the circle. When she did this a view would become visible through that circle. It was a view of fields and woods on a beautiful summer's day, a view into which she would feel herself being drawn.

By now the young lady had moved beyond all restrictions of logical reasoning and was beginning to experience a shift in consciousness. She was on the brink of moving from subconscious awareness to true spiritual awareness. It is at this point that true spiritual healing really comes into its own. This is where true spiritual love lifts another person free of emotional restrictions. Spiritually speaking, I had taken her beyond physical perception. I was now ready to reveal the true reason behind her childless marriage.

I asked her if she could see anything or anyone in the beauty she was now experiencing. She remained quiet for a long time (in these situations five minutes seems like an eternity). She then whispered that she could see a baby in the distance.

'Hold out your arms so it knows you want it,' I suggested.

'That won't solve anything,' she snapped. We now had a complete change of attitude. Gone was the calm, gentle woman; she had been replaced by a determined, though also frightened one.

'What won't it solve?' I asked.

'The baby will only come to replace me; the baby will take my place in Alec's affections. I will be left out. It will be Alec's baby.'

'Ask the baby why you haven't conceived to give it birth,' I continued.

Again after a long silence she said, 'Baby says he will not come while I feel he is coming for my husband's love and not mine. Baby says his love bond is with me and Alec will only be able to love him through me and he won't come until I fully acknowledge this.'

I then told her that when she could accept the truth of this statement to hold her arms out and let the spirit baby she could see and hear come to her for love. After a very long interval she opened her eyes which were full of tears. 'It was a beautiful experience,' she said, 'I held my baby.'

There was no need for her to come again and a few months later I received a lovely letter from her saying her baby was due in six months' time.

Every case of spiritual healing is unique, and unlike any other individual's experience, but the emotions it causes are always the same. These are spiritual emotions that can be experienced by everyone who has a problem, be it physical, emotional or spiritual, if only they learn to accept the truth of spiritual love and experience it through spiritual healing.

SPIRITUAL LOVE

For me spiritual healing means constantly making available the love which is my awareness to help another if they should have need of it. And what do I do with that love? Nothing. The love which I am is for others to make use of. It is not for me to limit or share what I am. Love just is. Love has no function, no purpose, in itself, but those who accept it without fear will become free of pain and disease as it rekindles the flame of their own love. As love increases, so the emotions of peace, happiness and contentment will grow in all who come into its sphere. But we can never know our own love until it is accepted by another and reflected back.

I am reminded of a woman I know who has a most difficult life. She has no husband, a child with terrible deformities, and no source of income except that which the State provides. This woman is shunned by most people because she smokes, swears and once a week, while a friend looks after her pitiful child, she goes out and drinks. People avoid her because they feel she is socially unacceptable, but to me she is an angel.

I know of no other living person who would love her poor deformed, slobbering child as she does. Her love pours out for her child and she has given everything she possesses to ensure that the child is loved and knows it is loved. So much love pours out of this woman that other children are drawn to her. You can see the love shine bright in their eyes for this woman who has nothing and does nothing except 'love'. Many people avoid or criticise, but to me she stands head and shoulders above them all — a beacon of love in a loveless society. It isn't what we do that is important; it is what we are.

In the same way spiritual love is not something you do; it is something you are. This is probably the most important sentence in the book, so take a few moments to think about it. There is no single act which demonstrates spiritual love. Love is intangible; those who are love will not be aware of it but others will. We can never know our own spirit, for love is like the light of a candle. It shines away from the centre and the one who is the cause of that light will never be aware of the love they radiate. So, what does light do? Nothing, it just is. But, like love, we can use it if we wish.

There are many who spend their lives doing wonderful unselfish acts of kindness, but even this isn't the love I speak of. The love I mean is not kindness but the essence of life itself which calls forth kindness in others. This love is the soul or spirit; it is God's expression on earth. To know and experience this love requires a change of perception for most people. It needs a shift in consciousness. It doesn't mean seeing, or hearing, or touching, or smelling, or tasting; it means becoming one with. To experience through the body is to experience life through the limits of mind and body. To experience through the spirit means becoming one with life itself.

I don't hear the sound of the wind rustling the leaves; I become one with the sound and I experience the sensations of the breeze as it jostles the leaves. That way I experience the music of sound. I don't watch the marvel of water playing over rocks in a stream; I become one with the water and flow with it to experience its movement. I don't touch a flower in the spring; I become one with the flower and know the meaning of its life. Love is not something you do; it is something you become, something you are. Love is not limited to time or place, or even dimension. It is beyond measurement. Love is Awareness of Love.

Love is not something you can give to another. Love is not something you can own or cultivate. Love is the essence of a spiritual existence. I don't get my ecstasy of life from myself; I can't know myself. My fulfilment comes from others, from their joy and happiness. And though I cannot give my love others can partake of it and become one with it. Spiritual love as spiritual awareness is a total experience.

To become one with nature means experiencing it and it is the greatest of experiences. Have you ever watched a bumble-bee? Next time you see one, try becoming one with it instead of watching it. Join with its thoughts as it buzzes here and there. To do this you must first be free of any thoughts of hurt or superiority. You must know that the love that you are is no greater than that of any other life or vision.

Then, as you marvel at the love which causes the bee to live you will find yourself being drawn to become one with it. Together, as equals, you will explore the flowers and the air, their scents and their music. Man is so superior that he hasn't even become equal to the bumble-bee. When you join with the sounds and sights of nature instead of listening and watching, you will have no need of intellect. You know God's mysteries without having to kill in order to learn.

The power of this kind of love is such that it lifts people out of their normal attitudes so that they begin to view life and death as a continuing process. Existence itself is perceived as being so great, so marvellous, that personal emotions are seen for what they are, just passing reactions to insignificant events. We come to realise and know that we are an insignificant part in some enormous happening but at the same time we can be one with the whole of that happening. The individual who has experienced this shift in consciousness loses sight of his own personality, his own growth, his own superiorities and insecurities. He comes to the realisation that all valued awareness is based on the radiated love we receive from other life. And it is this, and not the love which we radiate ourselves, that we experience. We are here for the benefit of others. We have no value for ourselves; we attract only that which we are.

Spiritual love, like spiritual healing, is something which can only be known by experiencing it. There are some for whom it is out of reach because they are not prepared to open themselves to a shift in consciousness or because they have a feeling of superiority. People such as these, who are unable to experience spiritual love, will continue to ridicule, scoff and criticise, as a way of overcoming their spiritual inadequacies.

To really experience and appreciate life, one needs to blend all the perceptions of pictures, sounds, smells, touches and tastes into one. This is probably best explained with light. If you break light down into its primary colours it becomes static, like a rainbow. To fully appreciate light, it needs to be seen as a mixture of colour and movement. Awareness is also moving, changing. It is about now. The past and the future are images and as such we can't be part of them. There is no spiritual awareness in a past or future reflection.

To achieve a shift in consciousness and know spiritual awareness is to become one with everything that is, and experience it. Then one's perception changes from watching to experiencing. One's ideas of God change from theories and philosophies to awareness. One becomes one with God, and one with every creation of loving thought, all at the same time. It is this total loving awareness which is the basis of spiritual healing. To know God is to abandon one's 'self' to become part of the totality of creative awareness.

People without spiritual awareness try to define God but how can you define that which you have not seen or experienced? Trying to define something with your current vocabulary is only using meaningless words to create the image of your own thoughts. It is impossible to define the totality of creative love with words. The only way to know God is to become one with the experience of God. The moment you stop to explain the emotions of that experience to another you lose spiritual awareness and are once again limited to words.

It is impossible to give someone the emotional experience of spiritual awareness by explaining it; just as a wedding photograph can't convey to someone who wasn't there the emotions of the occasion. Spiritual healing means helping another to reach their own spiritual awareness so that they can, themselves, become one with the wind, the river, the light and the unlimited love which is God. The closest I can get to describing the indescribable is to say that if you can see it or hear it you are not part of it and you can't truly understand it. As I said earlier, love is not something you do; it is something you are. To ask God to cure you of this or that is to completely miss the point. God doesn't do anything. God is. God doesn't heal you, any more than he causes you pain or despair. By opening yourself to a shift in consciousness, you heal yourself. God does not heal you. God is not this or that. God is total awareness, a spiritual experience. God is what you become when you learn how to give up and move from what you believe you are. The mountain cannot become one with a grain of sand but a grain of sand can become one with the mountain.

SPIRITUAL PURPOSE

The only value any of us have is what we can do for others. This is spiritual healing, using loving thoughts to benefit those around us. Negative individuals will take your energy anyway. Try and stop them and see what happens. You will become weaker as they take from you and, because you are deliberately not giving, you will not be creating more to replace that which is being taken.

This first became apparent to me very early on in my life. I remember having to go to the doctor's for something or other and opposite, lying in the arms of a very worried mother, was a baby. It couldn't have been very old, perhaps a month or two, and it looked terrible — pale, sick and lifeless. As I watched I felt my love for it growing and I felt that love being drawn from me in a most extraordinary way. It was as if something tangible was being extracted from my body. Not being sure what this was, I tried to stop it. I folded my arms, crossed my legs and tried to hold myself close, but it made little difference. This love, which was me, still kept going to the baby who needed it so much. After a while I began to feel totally drained and as I was obviously losing the battle to keep my strength to myself, I decided to give in gracefully and let it go without any selfish thoughts. I felt myself become one with the baby as it started to come to life. Colour returned to its cheeks, it started to kick and then pull faces and the resulting look of joy on its mother's face caused me to know the joy of love returned. Far from being exhausted I was actually exhilarated. I received far more than I had given because I had become one with another spirit of love.

Another lesson concerning love took place one hot summer's day. I had gone to the post office for a stamp. There was a long queue when I got there but my letter was urgent and so I had to join the queue. In front of me was a mother with a little girl of about seven or eight who had a large bouquet of wild flowers in her hand. When it was their turn to be served it quickly became clear that the mother was a talker. You know the sort I mean: loves to chat, thinks everyone is interested in her bunions, what the cat brought up last night, etc. Well she went on and on. Apparently they were on holiday,

'We haven't had a holiday in the country before,' she said and we all had to listen to a speech about how beautiful our fields and woods were, and how pretty our lanes were. ('Did she think we didn't know for heaven's sake? We did live there! All I wanted was a stamp.)

Then the little girl piped up,

'Oh no,' I thought, 'Not you as well.'

'I picked these flowers from the hedges,' she said, obviously very pleased with herself.

'You shouldn't pick our wild flowers,' I thought. 'It's against the law, go and put them back.'

By now people in the queue were beginning to shuffle so the post mistress, having decided there was no useful gossip to be had from this one, took her money and I moved forward. Mother and daughter went out of the shop completely unaware of the agitation they had caused. I bought my stamp, got to the door and then it hit me — a terrible feeling of guilt. They were only on holiday, probably their first. Why hadn't I wished them well and hoped they would have a wonderful week? Why hadn't I told the little girl how lovely her flowers looked? It would have cost me nothing and would have made their day even happier. I had withheld love that had been entrusted to me for another.

I felt sick, my stomach just seemed to turn over. True, they hadn't lost anything in love or happiness, but I could have given them so much more.

For weeks after that incident my stomach rolled over every time I thought about it. Eventually the illicitly held love burnt itself out and stopped hurting. But if such a seemingly trivial act of selfishness causes such a big pain what happens to those who have been horrendously selfish or destructive when the light of reason is eventually allowed to shine into their souls? If there is a hell that must be it — to have to face the destructive effects of one's own selfishness.

To use the forces of spirit and nature, or God if you prefer, you need to be totally free of the limitations of 'self-awareness'. You need to move beyond ordinary human expression or personality and become one with that greater awareness of Divine spiritual love. In this state there is no judgement, and there is no emotion other than the creative force of love. When you move, free of the body and into the ecstasy of unbounded love, you open up your vehicle, your body, to reach into the thoughts of another. Then if they choose, and only if they choose, they can use whatever love they possess to act as a link and replenish themselves from the energies you are making available.

Often at times of spiritual healing those receiving the love will break down and sob. This is not the release of trauma mentioned in earlier chapters; the reactions and responses are totally different. There can never be any doubt when the healing is spiritual but unless you have experienced it you cannot comprehend the majesty of it. In all this the healer has to be totally free of physical emotion in order to join with forces which cannot recognise hate, envy, selfishness, etc.

———————— *NEGATIVE EMOTIONS* ————————

I am often asked if I ever protect myself from the bad thoughts or emotions of others. Many people seem to think that this is necessary, but why? If your thoughts are totally of love then any thoughts not of love are hardly likely to blend with yours. In order to help people in emotional or spiritual pain it's necessary to become one with them.

It's quite simple when you remember that in essence we are only spirit anyway and joining with one body is not too unlike joining with another. How can you possibly help someone who is full of hate and anger if you don't get inside with him and find out what's caused his problem for yourself. Believe me, if you learn how to experience another's thoughts and actions in this way you won't ever judge anyone again. From the outside we can never know what has caused another to be as they are. And when we get inside and become one with their deeper emotions, can we honestly say we would have acted differently?

When someone comes for help full of hate and anger, jealousy or hurt, I need to know what caused it. What they tell me caused it, and what I experience as their reason for being that way, are usually very different. As a healer my first step is to help them convert the anger or hurt into more creative energy. Hate is energy (just as love is energy) but it is misused energy. So I take to myself all the hate and anger which they care to throw out. If you don't allow someone to express and rid themselves of their anger it will keep on increasing.

I was once a salesman and whenever I had a nasty situation to defuse, such as an irate customer who felt he had cause to complain, I would wait until he had vented all his anger and then take out a notebook and pencil and say, 'Yes sir, I can see you have a reason for complaining. Would you please repeat what you have just said exactly, word for word, including the adjectives, so that I can give a copy to my boss.' Then I would wait. Have you ever seen anyone try and repeat something said in anger if they have been allowed to finish and fully expose their emotions? Once all the anger had been used up they can't repeat it, no matter how hard they try.

If you ask them to repeat it so that you can write it down they will probably try once or twice to remember what it was they said. But, in trying to remember why they were so angry it will begin to sound foolish even to them. Usually they stop looking belligerent and even begin to grin or laugh. But what would have happened if I hadn't let him finish? If I had reacted with anger or argued or just walked away he would have become even more annoyed and we would have parted, each leaving the other even angrier than before we began.

Sometimes, of course, the anger or resentment is so deep, so intense, that it takes many, many sessions before it is all released and those standing in its way will feel they can take no more. But as long as they don't allow themselves to become emotionally involved and negative in their attitude towards the situation, another's negative emotions will not affect them. If someone needs to vent their anger and frustration towards me, at me, or in my presence, I would not be helping either of us if I tried to prevent it or walked away. I suppose this is what is meant by 'turning the other cheek'.

In some instances the anger and resentment seem to increase if the healer just stands there and says nothing, because the vindictive are hoping for a reaction, a retort, on which they can build further anger. Provided the one absorbing the negative attitudes does nothing, but continues to soak it all up, even if it takes hours, days, weeks or years, the one suffering from hurt will eventually have spent all their frustration. Then love will fill the void, and that is spiritual healing.

ABSENT HEALING

I am constantly called on to heal others who are at a distance from me. This is called absent healing, and those who have experienced a shift in consciousness will have no difficulty understanding this and being able to receive another's healing energies in this way. When someone receives spiritual love as healing, they will experience freedom from pain or hurt which always become less as fear disappears. Again I must emphasise that I can only explain what it is like for me as a healer, for the ways of other spiritual healers may well be different from mine.

I can only say that I don't feel as if I'm part of my body or mind. Instead I exist away from it, using my body merely as a vehicle for communication. As spirit I exist through all time and space, and through all dimensions. I know of no boundaries in the eternity of love. I know this might sound strange, and people say to me, 'How can you possibly be in all places at the same time?'

I answer, 'How can you possibly stay limited within the space of a body?'

It is because I know myself to be in all places at the same time that absent healing is so natural for me. Let me try and explain. When you speak, your words travel out in all directions; they can be heard above and below, in front and behind, all at the same time. But no matter where your words are heard, they are still part of you. Your words do not cease to be you because they are no longer on your lips. It is the same with your thoughts which, once expressed, exist forever.

When your body has ceased to house you, and you experience death, all you are left with are your thoughts. You are the sum total of your thoughts at any one time and they travel out from the centre of the spirit. But there can be no centre to something which is fluid because radiating perception can be in any place. Spirit has no organisational centre like the brain (which the body uses to organise physical perceptions). If someone across the oceans asks, with their thoughts, for you to heal them, your love is immediately aware of it.

The difference between spiritual healing and what I term physical healing is that one needs no contact and can be conducted from the other side of the world, while the other needs close if not direct contact. All spiritual healing is really absent healing. As it implies, absent healing means that the one being treated need not necessarily be in the vicinity of the healer.

The difference between the two types of healing is quite fundamental. Physical healing works directly upon the body or the mind controlling the body. It is physical or emotional energy, in the form of electromagnetic fields, giving direct physical help to another. Spiritual healing uses the strength of love as a non-quantifiable energy to make it possible for another to heal himself, spiritually, physically and emotionally. The reason that distance is no barrier to spiritual healing is that distance is no barrier to spiritual activity.

Our spiritual thoughts travel out into time and space to affect, if accepted, other similar thought forms. Everything that exists vibrates, and has its own electromagnetic field which vibrates into space to be received by anything in harmony with it. It's just like receiving a radio signal. Some of my most profound healing successes have been due to absent healing. Strangely enough, two of them were very similar, both brain tumours.

The first was in about 1984. A very good friend of ours was working in London and she started having bad headaches. Sue went to see a consultant who confirmed that she had a brain tumour, but after a course of radiotherapy the pain and the tumour still persisted. Eventually she was told that her life expectancy was no more than three months. The woman in question, who was forty-three and a secretary to a company director, decided to continue working for as long as possible.

At that point she asked for my help.

I met her in London and as I passed my hand over her head she screamed out with pain. She explained that it was as if someone had put a red-hot needle through her brain. I told her to phone me whenever she had a pain but, apart from that, there was no need for further contact and I would send her absent healing. This only works when there is a close harmony or trust between recipient and healer. It is less successful when the trust is not total and the spirit of the one needing help not fully in tune with the thoughts of the healer.

During the following weeks she phoned several times with a headache, usually from work. I would ask her to lock herself in her office and sit quietly and concentrate on me for half an hour. At the end of that time I told her to phone me to confirm that the pain had gone. I would then sit quietly and concentrate on my friend. The three months came and went. She had by now stopped going to the hospital because there was nothing more they could do except offer her pain-killers. After five months she needed no more treatment from me. By that time I had already told her that the tumour had gone and the hospital then confirmed it. During the whole of that period we had not seen each other since the first meeting in London.

Another very similar case involved a woman from the Channel Islands. I had been to see a friend and while I was with her she told me that she had been getting headaches behind one eye for several weeks. I gave her healing to remove the headache but explained that she had nothing physically wrong and that the pain was due to someone else's illness.

A few days later my friend telephoned to say that her sister, whom I shall refer to as Helen, had just been admitted to hospital with a confirmed growth on her pituitary gland. Helen had not been having headaches and the symptoms had only started a few days earlier when the sight in her left eye had begun to become obscured. Having seen an optician on the Friday and then an eye surgeon on the Saturday, she had been referred to an eye hospital on the Monday. She was examined and immediately sent on to a neurological hospital where she was formally admitted on the Wednesday. It was decided that an operation would be necessary but because it was only a few days before Christmas the operation was put back until January.

During the Christmas holiday Helen was able to visit me for a single treatment. After that all the healing was absent healing. I told her that I was sure the hospital would have no need to go ahead with the operation because the absent healing would cause the tumour to go away.

On the Monday a week or two later Helen was admitted to hospital and given a scan the same afternoon. Her operation had been arranged to take place on Wednesday. Much to the surgeon's amazement the scan showed no trace of the growth. Neither was any scar tissue visible though the growth had shown up clearly on earlier scans taken in December on two separate occasions. The healing had clearly been successful.

Helen became the subject of a discussion at the hospital and many specialists were there at the case conference to hear the details and discuss it. They were not told that Helen had been receiving absent healing. Helen was present on stage during the talk and at the end of the discussion one of the doctors asked what her opinion was of the remarkable cure. She told him quite plainly that she had no doubts that it was due to spiritual healing. With this remark total quiet descended on the audience and they quickly hurried on to the next subject.

It is also worth noting that at exactly the same time that I was treating Helen in my clinic her sister's headaches disappeared and they have not returned. Helen was repeatedly asked by the doctors if she was getting headaches but she had never had one.

On the only occasion when Helen had visited me for healing, her husband, who was present in the room, developed a 'blinding' headache which I treated, though at no time did Helen have a headache. Her eyesight is now almost completely recovered, although in certain lights there is still a blind spot in one eye. This has been put down to the growth having 'frayed' a small part of the optic nerve.

As an aside, when I asked for permission to add this story to the book Helen's husband suggested that I include the fact that at the time Helen had been admitted to the hospital for the first tests he had been terribly worried. Then he suddenly realised that everything would be all right. He says it was an amazing feeling. He later found out that this great sense of calm came upon him at the same time that Helen's sister had telephoned me to ask if I would send absent healing.

Absent healing is a very potent force. I use it in all sorts of situations. I have been with people, in a spiritual sense, at funerals to give them strength and support, and at interviews to give confidence, as well as the usual absent healing situations. Many times I have had it confirmed that the one receiving the absent healing had known I was there because they phone and tell me that friends who were with them experienced it as well. The problem with all this is that it is impossible to prove and the sceptics prefer to laugh and ridicule — that is until they themselves need the help which can only come from a healer.

I can't prove that any of the healing that comes from absent healing is due to me. Neither can any other healer. We know and we just have to leave it at that. Knowing for ourselves is what is important, not proving it. How do you prove to someone born blind that there is a sunset or a sunrise or explain the beauty of poppies in a cornfield? How do you prove to someone born deaf that there is beauty in the sound of water bubbling over rocks or a skylark singing? I can't prove to you, or anyone else, the experiences I have when I'm free of the shell which is my body.

HEALING TO RELEASE LIFE

As a healer it's not always my purpose to sustain life. This may sound very odd but it's happened to me so often that now I just accept it. The first time this was made apparent was right at the start of my entry into healing. In those early days, before I was so busy, I would quite willingly travel across counties to see people if asked to do so. I had received a phone call from a lady about 80 miles away. Would I please go and help her husband who was dying of lung cancer. My wife and I set off and when we were within 5 miles of our destination we had to phone for clearer instructions because we were looking for a little village somewhere in the country.

'I'm sorry I asked you to come,' she said, 'but the doctor has just been and doesn't expect John to survive another hour. I'm afraid it's all too late.'

'Having come this far, can we just call and meet you anyway?' I asked. And so a few minutes later we were in their front room in which a single bed had been put in for John. He looked ghastly — unconscious and as ill as you would expect from the doctor's prognosis. While John's wife Mary was making a cup of tea I went across and put my hand over his head, then over his heart and again, after about fifteen minutes, over his head. After about twenty minutes he opened his eyes, in another ten minutes he was propped fully up and half an hour after that he was having a cup of tea and talking. The doctor called in again and was stunned. Naturally we were all delighted, eventually leaving but promising to call back next week.

It was exactly the same scene the following week. John was again close to death, unconscious, with the doctor calling, expecting the worst in a few hours' time. Apparently John had been remarkable, considering his condition, for the first part of the week but he had gradually slipped back to the state he was now in. I went through the healing performance again with exactly the same result. John was drinking tea when we drove away. The following week was exactly the same — John dying, only to be brought back for another week of pain for him, and despair for his wife. This couldn't go on. I was interfering in a natural process, a person's right to return home when they had been called. It might sound terrible but I deliberately found excuses not to go the next week and he died on the day I would have been there. All I had done in the preceding weeks was delay the inevitable, causing prolonged pain and suffering to both husband and wife. I don't have the right, spiritual or otherwise, to decide who lives and who dies.

Many times I have helped people move from this world to the next. I recall one particular situation. A woman — lets call her Jean, phoned and asked if I would call. Jean had a particularly nasty lung cancer, which would, she told me, spread very slowly through her lungs and eventually choke her. Around her bed were bottles of oxygen which she used from time to time when her need was desperate. She was about fifty-five and had been told that she would live for about six months — a terrible fate. I called every other day for a week. I knew from the beginning that I wasn't going to alter the situation, but I did seem to give her comfort and ease her distress. After a few visits she asked directly, 'Do you think you can cure me?'

I answered by saying, 'I don't cure anyone. I just give whatever it is I have to help people to heal themselves. It is God who decides if you stay here or move on to the next world.' Then I asked if she prayed.

She said that she did.

'Then why don't you ask Him?'

I suggested that that evening when she said her prayers, she should say to God: 'If it is Your intention that I come home to You I accept that with love and understanding. Also if it is Your will that I am to remain here, even as an invalid, I accept that too with love and understanding. But please don't leave me without an answer. Give me a sign of what you intend and want of me.'

I hadn't intended to return for two days, but the next day I received a phone call from her son asking me to go right away. When I got there she was struggling for breath and the family were expecting the worst, even though the doctor had visited the day before and confirmed that Jean still had six months left. I sat on the bed beside her.

'Why are they all crying?' she asked as she looked at her relatives around the room.

'They are upset because of the pain you must be suffering,' I said.

'But I haven't got any pain,' she answered, looking very puzzled by the reason I had given.

This was from a lady struggling to breathe, and gasping as

if her lungs were in agony.

'Am I dying?' she asked,

'Did you ask God for an answer as we discussed?' I returned.

She gave me a lovely smile, 'Yes, I did,' she said.

'Then you are getting your answer, aren't you?'

With that she closed her eyes and went to sleep. About five minutes later I saw her spirit lift from her body. She gave me the most beautiful smile I have ever seen and with that she just floated away. The now empty shell still seemed as before, alive and breathing, only I knew that it was now empty of life. But it still had sufficient energy to continue living for a while on its own. I went downstairs and waited. It was a full half hour before I heard cries of grief from the room above indicating that the body had come to its end.

Now when I am asked to see someone who is terminally ill I don't have any preconceived ideas about what I'm going for. I just go with the intention of releasing whatever it is I am asked to release and doing what has to be done. Many times I'm told, 'You didn't come on your own. Someone came in with you. I can feel and see their presence.'

Very often that someone takes back to the next world the one I've gone to see. Dying is so easy, provided it is free of fear. A doctor's prognosis is very often wrong and I wouldn't just lie down and die because it was expected of me. But if I were certain that the physical body couldn't survive, for whatever reason, I would accept it. No one would ever be able to say of me that 'He didn't give in easily.' I really don't see the point of trying to stay with a body that's rejecting you. If your time has come to go back to the other dimension, then you will go, if not today — eagerly and accepting release — then tomorrow after a terrific struggle which is only going to prolong the agony.

When my time comes I shall be off. I shan't wait for my body to disintegrate and for me to experience all its falling apart before I go. I've seen too many people fight and the suffering they bring upon themselves in the final struggle is awful to watch. I've also seen those who accept death with dignity, those who know of the better experience to come. Their attitudes and emotions are totally different, as they slip into death and out of their shell.

I really do think it is barbaric trying to keep someone alive against the odds with drugs. The only real responsibility we have for those whose time is close at hand is to administer love, and when that is not sufficient to keep them with us and pain-free they will go peacefully. That does not mean I am against pain-killers or any other form of treatment. But, for example, to use drugs to keep old people alive when they are in pain, on their own and probably not even mentally aware, is I believe inhuman. Usually the spirit of such people has already departed and the doctors are just fighting to keep a corpse breathing. This is not a criticism of doctors, who do what needs to be done. It is the system and culture we live in which is wrong.

For instance, I have a friend whose elderly mother was over ninety. She was living out her existence in a nursing home. She wasn't safe around the house and needed constant care. She was doubly incontinent, had a diseased hip which gave constant pain, had lost her memory so that she couldn't remember one day to the next, and had a life that was restricted to one small room. She was unable to read, watch television or hold a sensible conversation. She just wanted to die, to 'go back home' as she used to say.

Then she caught a cold which turned to pneumonia, a quiet and peaceful way to pass from this world. But no, the doctor gave her antibiotics, against the family's wishes, and she recovered. This happened several times and she lived through another four years of misery. I can understand the doctor's actions. He would have been acting unlawfully if he had done anything else. These cases put doctors in an awful position but it does seem unnatural to prolong life in this sort of situation. Healing does much more than keep people alive or free them from pain or physical injury. It gives the spirit freedom to return home with its dignity intact if its time has come.

Some will be asking how I can possibly know this. One reason is that on many occasions those who have left their shell return to me with messages of thanks and personal accounts of what it's like in the next world.

One such experience concerned a lady who had died of cancer. A few days after she had passed to the next world she returned. Gone was the tired and exhausted look of pain, instead before me was a beautiful expression of love in shimmering white. Recognition was through the eyes. She told me of the beauty and peace she had gone back to, of the overwhelming love she was now part of. She told me that dying and leaving her body had been so easy that if she could avoid being born she would do it all over again. Sometimes the dying have such a fear of returning to the next world that instead of allowing themselves to be taken back they just remain in this dimension. Some people are terrified of what awaits us. Usually because of the religions they have been brought up in damnation serves its purpose in preventing the freed spirit from returning home.

One particular case I remember concerned a young girl of about thirteen. I had been asked to exorcise a ghost or presence in an old manor house. Apparently there was a presence in the kitchen which was causing a lot of concern amongst the staff. The presence was recognised by a cold sensation which moved around the room, sometimes a presence was visible, but only as an electrical discharge. I went into the kitchen and in a spiritual sense made contact with a young girl who told me she had once worked in the kitchen and felt secure there. She had died young but instead of moving into a light which she could see, as she had been instructed to do after leaving her body, she stayed where she was because she believed she was destined to go to hell. She had at some time in her young life been naughty and was told naughty girls go to hell. To her that meant all sorts of terrifying ordeals and so great was the emotion of fear that she couldn't break free of it and so stayed in this dimension. I was able to help by giving her the confidence to make the transition to a world of love. The atmosphere in the kitchen then returned to normal.

In these situations I have been called upon many times to help people die and travel on to the new dimension. I sometimes travel, in spirit, with these people. Because they know me and trust me they will begin the journey with me. As I explained earlier in the book, I am not of my body. Because I am spiritually aware of this, those who have returned to spiritual awareness allow me to help them so that together we can move forward into a world that is felt rather than seen. The beauty, peace and love we travel through is truly overwhelming and when this love has engulfed the spirit I'm helping, others come and take over from me. If everyone could experience such an event just once in their lives it would change the world.

— 8 —

Ejecting

There is often a lot of confusion between the terms 'spiritual' and 'spiritualism'. Spiritual means 'from God', 'God-given', 'with God's love'. Spiritual, as applied to healing, means 'with God's love' whereas spiritualism is a philosophy or belief that the spirits of the dead can and do communicate with the living. I have no argument with this, and many spiritualists are very good healers. I owe my beginnings as a healer to the encouragement and help I received from the spiritualist movement, though I do not practise spiritualism. Spiritualists are those who have experienced a shift in consciousness or who have always had spirit perception as well as physical perception.

—————— SPIRITUALISM ——————

Modern spiritualism can be traced back to 1848 and an old cottage in Hydesville, New York. The cottage had been haunted for some time by various poltergeist sounds and movements, particularly a banging noise during the night. The little girl who lived there, Katie Fox, far from being frightened, began to play a game with the bumps and sounds of the night by bumping back. She soon found that she was getting some sort of intelligent response and so worked out a simple code and began conversing with the mysterious visitor. I suppose it could be claimed that she invented the ouija board.

The messages she got from the unseen visitor told her that he had been a pedlar and he had been murdered in the cottage and was now demanding a decent burial. Not much seems to have been done about the pedlar but some remains are said to have been found under the cellar floor. Word soon got around and crowds began to gather in great numbers and soon it seemed that there were as many visitors to the cottage from the next dimension as there were in this one. Katie and her sisters eventually moved to the nearby city where they spent their lives as mediums.

Soon mediums began popping up all over America and there was never a shortage of departed spirits wanting talk to them. The spiritualist movement had arrived, and with it a whole new philosophy about what happens to the spirit once it is free of the body. Of course none of this was new. The Egyptians were far more sophisticated in the way that they communicated with the dead and their high priests are said to have possessed knowledge which allowed them to travel independently of their bodies.

Perhaps I should make my position on all this quite clear. I accept, not as faith but as fact, that we can and do leave our bodies. I believe that my body is something I use, not something I am. Life does exist after death and we can communicate with some of the departed. Whether we should is another question.

After the first 300 hundred years of Christianity the church decided to drive out all opposition to its own authority, even to the point of denying the very principles upon which it was founded. Some of these principles are that there is life after death, that departed spirits can and do guide and assist us in our lives on earth, that dying and departing is a simple matter, that provided one uses the love of one's spirit anyone can heal, and that healing each other is a necessary human activity.

The early Christian leaders were all healers and mediums

(i.e. prophets) but when King Constantine took over as leader of the Christian church in AD 312 he chose as his advisers people whose gifts were no greater than his own. As he had no gifts himself it was only a matter of time before anyone with spiritual gifts was considered a threat to his authority and subjected to ridicule or worse. Ceremony and superiority took the place of spiritual gifts and equality. And when it is remembered that King Constantine was a pagan sun worshipper until the last few hours of his life it is hardly surprising.

Therefore the revival of a belief in the supernatural has been seen as a direct threat to orthodox religion which is based on dogma. Over the years the church desperately tried to suppress spiritualism, but to no avail as spiritualism gave people hope of a future and answers to questions which the church couldn't give. Very late in the day, when the church realised that a lot of good was coming from spiritualist healing, it began to accept and offer 'faith healing' as if it alone had discovered it and it alone had the authority to use it, while still opposing those who had reintroduced the idea.

Because of all this, we now have a silly situation whereby many orthodox religions are saying that all healing should be done under their supervision; and if practised by others, they say, the healing may not be genuine and could even be dangerous. We also have all sorts of 'New Age' religions springing up as offshoots of spiritualism. These are really anything but 'new' (most of them are Celtic in origin). We have various Eastern and Oriental philosophies attracting a large following, as well as many evangelical organisations and groups which are all variations on the original Christian church. Each one believes that it alone holds God's confidence and loyalty; that all the others are misleading in some way and probably doing their followers terrible spiritual harm.

Personally I don't think it matters what your personal philosophy is. No two people are alike and each must choose that moral philosophy which best allows them to mature spiritually and help others, whenever requested to do so. My own views are quite simple. I believe in a single God, as a creative, loving force. I believe that He communicates with the world through the beauty of His creations, and that we communicate with Him with the love we pass on through the lives of others. It's as simple as that. For me, the ceremony and superiority of many organised religions take the faith out of believing and knowing.

—— OUT-OF-BODY EXPERIENCES (OBE) ——

Many people have had an OBE. To some it is a frightening experience, not to be repeated. To others it is a wonderful experience. It's something I find quite natural and it's the state I assume when I'm healing.

It's like driving a car. How often do you travel somewhere but find that you cannot recall a part of the journey? The brain, or computer, has been programmed to drive for you. And provided the computer is not confronted by a situation it has not previously experienced, it will drive the car perfectly well without your being aware of the journey. You, the spirit, will be somewhere else. This, of course, is not a complete OBE but for those who haven't experienced one it will give some idea of the mechanics.

As I explained earlier we are electronically sealed into our body which has been our experience of life over the preceding years. As long as the flow of electromagnetic energy is maintained there is no way we can easily experience life 'body-free'. However if we could reduce the energy flow then the magnetic grip which the body's energy has over us would be lessened and we would remember a few minutes of our out-of-body experiences.

A typical example of this is when an anaesthetist reduces brainwave activity too far during an operation and the patient finds himself floating on the ceiling, or somewhere else, watching his own operation. As the anaesthetic wears off, and brain activity increases, the spirit is quickly pulled back to the original state. At the end of life, when the brain is becoming less efficient at generating energy we will begin to experience that floating feeling. Eventually, when brain functions stop completely and our energy flow is halted we simply float free of our bodies to resume life where we left it before we came to the earth-physical dimension.

In any situation where a person's energy is below the level required to bind them to their body they may experience the beginnings of an OBE. The first symptom of such an experience is usually a feeling of floating and feeling light-headed. Sometimes people tell me they feel as though they are falling out of their bodies; in some extreme situations people actually experience a few moments watching themselves from outside as if their own body belonged to another person.

The most bizarre case of this that I can remember was a woman who came to me because she thought she was going mad. She kept seeing herself from other parts of the room. This particular woman had problems in just about every area of her life. She had an alcoholic husband, financial worries, personal health problems, delinquent children and elderly parents. No wonder her energy levels were depleted. She was using huge quantities of energy in personal worry and ill-health; her surrounding family were also draining her of all the energy they could get. In this situation energy levels were bound to drop; indeed they dropped so low that her body lost its magnetic hold over her spirit and she began to drift away from her body.

Often when people are just falling asleep or just waking they feel as if they are not properly in their bodies. While we are sleeping our energy, or brainwave activity, is at its lowest, and many people experience an OBE during the night. But as long as the brain keeps ticking over, the magnetic link between spirit and body continues to exist. The moment the brain becomes active, the energy levels will rise and the spirit is pulled back into its body.

People who have experienced an OBE tell of a silver cord

which seems to connect them to their body. This silver cord is the electrical current, or magnetic energy which continues to attract the spirit until, for whatever reason, the current is broken. At this point we become totally separated from our bodies in death. I have no doubt that it is absolutely pain free because I have seen people die and their spirit rise from their body. In one instance it was several hours after the spirit had gone that the body actually expired and the spirit became free to return to other dimensions.

Some people are capable of deliberately reducing their energy levels by fasting and starving so that their electronic lock is weakened, allowing them to have an OBE. Certain gurus, fakirs and other mystics seem to find some satisfaction from behaving unnaturally in this way. I personally believe that we have a responsibility to experience this life and learn to conquer its selfishness and fear rather than set ourselves apart by abandoning current reality as if this signified some form of excellence.

This practice is not to be confused with meditation which is quite different. In meditation the mind is stilled in such a way that physical awareness travels inwards to see and experience some of the impressions of the spirit which is using the body. In other words the spirit uses the mind to look into its own thoughts. Using its physical and mental powers to reflect to physical consciousness the image of itself is nearly always deeply relaxing, as one is hardly likely to find thoughts that are out of harmony. Meditation is the art of looking into the spirit of oneself ('going-in'), whereas OBE is the art of being free of the physical shell and looking out.

EXTRA-PHYSICAL PERCEPTION (EPP)

One of the stranger aspects of spiritual healing is the ability of some healers to become one with the thoughts of a patient in such a way that the healer can experience their pains or emotions through his own body. I often use this technique to locate exactly where the problem is. It's quite easy really. As I have said I don't work *from* my own body, but *through* it, and when I'm healing I become one with the thoughts of the other. I feel what the patient feels by registering their pain, which my spirit feeds through to my own body. This is very difficult to comprehend if you haven't any spiritual perception, so I will give an example.

A woman had booked to come and see me. Her main problem, she said, was a general feeling of depression. There was no particular reason for it; she just felt ill. So she came, sat in the chair and we went through the normal routine of healing. After about ten minutes I began to feel the most awful pain in the area of my liver. I knew that there was nothing wrong with my liver so it had to be the patient's. At this point I went into a much deeper spiritual concentration by releasing myself from my own emotions. After about five minutes I knew what I needed to know.

'You didn't really come because of depression, did you?' I ventured. 'You think you have cancer of the liver and are hoping I will confirm it one way or the other and treat it for you if it is cancer. You have a pain right there, don't you?' I said, sticking a finger into the area where the liver is.

'Yes, that's right,' she said. 'How did you know?'

'Because I can feel your pain for myself. The intensity of your thoughts and pain are getting through to me and also spiritually you told me all about it just a few minutes ago.'

'Is it cancer?' This was her moment of truth.

'No.'

'Thank God for that,' she said.

'It's not even your pain. There is absolutely nothing wrong with you or your liver.'

'Well why am I getting this awful pain?'

'Has your husband been unwell?'

'Yes, but how do you know?'

'Spiritually you have just told me that the pain isn't yours.

It's your husband's pain which, because of the closeness between you both, you are experiencing for him.'

'What about my pain?' She was obviously wondering if she would have to continue suffering with him.

'Now you know the cause of the pain you won't experience it any more,' I said. 'In exactly the same way, as soon as I had worked out what was troubling you, the pain I was experiencing went.'

The woman then confirmed that she had been to the doctor the previous week for tests and was waiting for the results. When she got them they proved negative.

Many clients who come for treatment only tell me about the pain which is causing them the greater problem. Whenever a client does this I will sooner or later pick up on the pain I haven't been told about. This is particularly useful when a client's pain is a referred pain because then I will experience the pain at the site of the problem and this may be at a totally different place from where the client feels it.

My ability to do this can be a bit inconvenient at social gatherings though, particularly if someone there is unwell but has said nothing about it. I often pick up on other people's aches and pains and know before they do if they have unsuspected problems. I try to avoid it but it isn't always possible especially if I'm in a meditative frame of mind. I particularly dislike shopping in busy places for this very reason. Walking through a shop full of people can leave me physically and mentally drained. I pick up all the physical and emotional problems of the people I'm closest to and I automatically release energy as I pass or stand near them.

I particularly recall one situation which involved a mother and her daughter. The mother had stomach cancer and it had progressed a long way before it was discovered. The daughter who was in her thirties brought her mother to see me and explained that it was only weight loss and a feeling of exhaustion that had caused her mother to go to the doctor's for an examination at all. She went on to say that at no time had she even had pain.

I proceeded to give healing in the usual way and was instantly taken with stomach pains. But they were coming from the daughter rather than her mother. I asked the daughter if she had any pain and she admitted that she had. In fact she had had severe stomach pains for about nine months and the doctor hadn't been able to find anything wrong. He wasn't likely to, because the daughter, who was very spiritually close to her mother, wasn't ill. She was taking the pain for her mother, although she hadn't realised it. She hadn't said anything about her pains because she didn't want to upset anyone, especially as her mother was so ill and the doctor had confirmed that she herself had nothing to worry about.

I have also known children, especially girls, who have complained of pains for which no illness or injury could be diagnosed. I know of one poor lass who was always complaining of aches and pains somewhere or other. Eventually her family just ignored the girl's anguish, believing she was exaggerating or making it all up. But when I investigated it thoroughly I found that she was experiencing pain for other members of her family. In fact it had become a family joke. 'If anyone gets a headache or sore finger you can be sure Jill will get it as well,' they said. But it wasn't a joke to Jill who really was suffering. When I explained to her what was happening she was able to identify whose pain it was and distance herself from it.

Many people are spiritually in tune with those around them but they don't appreciate or understand what is going on. This is especially true of women who frequently experience pains for other members of the family.

ACCOUNTABILITY

I am often asked how I cope with all the unhappiness and pain I see. The truth is that it doesn't affect me with sadness at all. It is true that people from all walks of life come to me with all sorts of problem, asking for help. Often the only help I can give is love to quieten their fears. But one thing I never feel is sadness for them. I never feel pity or sympathy. These people already have all the unhappiness they can bear; they don't want me adding to it. They don't come to me so I can make them even more aware of their problems. They come to me in order to join in my peace, love and contentment, which helps them overcome their fear and pain. I never feel sorry for anyone. That may sound like an awful thing to say, but it's true. They are surrounded by people who feel sorry for them and what good does it do? They want love and understanding to lift them into a feeling of peace and contentment. You see, the emotions of pity and sympathy don't heal; they are negative, not positive.

Healers accept that positive, loving thoughts are the basis of absent healing. The religious pray for help and healing of the sick and they know their prayers are answered. This is exactly what the healer does with his healing thoughts and prayers. Therefore, if positive thoughts for the good of others will benefit them, is it not also logical to accept that negative or worrying thoughts will achieve the exact opposite? This is especially likely as negative and worrying thoughts are usually continuous, whereas positive healing thoughts are normally only in the mind for the duration of the prayer.

It is surprising how even those who send out prayers and absent healing for the well-being of others will spend time worrying about themselves and their families. Many people forget that any strong thoughts create an effect on those towards whom they are directed. When it is done positively with good intent the effect is beneficial. When the thought is negative, worrying or with negative concern, then the effect can be very damaging. How often parents worry about the health of their children, or children about the health of their parents. It may be done with love, but can they not see that these negative thoughts only deepen the problem instead of solving it? Can they not see that they are only adding to the pain already felt by those who are suffering?

Whole nations grieve and worry about the state of people living in warring countries. These are negative thoughts which do no good. Television commentators are full of negative news, causing millions of people to worry about the weather, their health, the environment. Negative thoughts such as these do nothing to counter the deprivation, pain and other difficulties suffered by the world's peoples. It's positive, loving thoughts that individuals, families, communities and nations need. Stop worrying about your children. Instead think of them lovingly. Your worry will change nothing, it will only add to their problems. All absent healing, all prayers, are based on the positive love of one being transferred to another in need, whether it be an individual or a nation.

This brings us to the point. Who is responsible for the healing power? God, some angel or guiding spirit or oneself? As we saw in the first part of the book, the body is a huge battery which produces electricity. It uses this energy to keep itself in good repair and it often has a surplus which others can use. This is becoming known as the science of bioelectricity and has nothing to do with God, spirits or anything of a metaphysical nature. Much of the healing we see today can be put into that category.

Spiritual healing is different. It is a power latent in every spirit and usually more readily found in the positive types than the negative. We are all responsible for allowing the love which has been gifted to us to aid others. The love, or light or spiritual energy which a healer uses for absent healing is their own. It has been gifted to them by God. But they cannot stand aside and say that God has healed through them, relinquishing all responsibility for what was taking place.

If God wanted to heal without making man responsible for what he does, He would. It makes no sense to believe that the Universal Spirit whom we call God needs anyone to help Him achieve anything. The Universal Spirit prefers to give opportunity to those who want to use the love of their souls to help others. Healers may be guided and fuelled by the Master Creator but healers decide for themselves if and when their spiritual love will be used. That does not mean that healers will always be successful. Sometimes they take on tasks which are too great for their limited powers; sometimes the patients don't trust or open their spirit to the healing powers because of lack of harmony between healer and client. It's not succeeding that is important, it's trying to succeed and recognising one's own limitations.

The spirits that some healers feel are with them may be spirit guides, those who help us through life. If we allow them to, these spirit guides will help us with spiritual development in many ways, including healing. Spirit guides are personalities of a higher dimension whose love and wisdom is such that they are able to help us through difficult and trying times. But we have lived many times in ages past and every life gives us a fresh personality, a different experience. Many of the personalities we feel around us are in fact facets of our own greater personality developed in previous lives. This brings us neatly to another type of healing, 'reincarnation healing'.

— 9 —

The Parachute Opens

REINCARNATION

Reincarnation is the doctrine that spirits experience more than one life on earth, and that each life adds to the overall personality of the spirit as it slowly evolves through the ages. Belief in reincarnation goes back to pre-biblical times. It was the basis of Christianity and was only declared a heresy by the Second Christian Council of Constantinople in AD 553. Prior to that, reincarnation was widely accepted. It was taught by the Gnostics and Essenes with whom Jesus spent his early years. In fact Jesus reincarnated to give proof of life after death. Most of the early civilisations accepted reincarnation, especially those which placed a high value on esoteric thinking such as the Celtic Druids, American Indians, and other spiritual peoples of the world. It was also part of Plato's thinking.

The different theories of reincarnation and the data supporting its theories would take another book and anyway there are already plenty on the market. But reincarnation does touch on the fringes of healing and is often used by the sceptics to discredit the whole healing philosophy, so it is worth discussing it in some detail.

Materialistic, Western thinkers find it difficult to accept the principle of reincarnation. This could be because they believe that one life on earth should be enough for anyone or because their minds are not yet ready to conceive of the enormous consequences of an evolving spirit journeying through time, space and different dimensions, often repeating the more difficult parts of the journey to correct past mistakes or learn new lessons. All I know is that personally I have no difficulty accepting the reincarnation principle after a series of very inspiring experiences. Just in case it crosses your mind at this point, I should mention that I do not take drugs and never have taken them. I rarely drink alcohol and have never been drunk, so I have to accept these experiences for what they were.

Leaving my body or thinking independently of it allows me to see the world to come. It also means that I can use perception not normally available to those stuck in a pilot's cockpit. Believe me, life before life is a fact, the only reason you don't remember anything about it is that while in the body you have to use the facilities of the body. That includes the memory and its database and this physical apparatus has no memory or information predating its own existence. Therefore while stuck in the body your perception of time and life, dimension and existence is restricted to what you have experienced since conception or shortly after. Those of us, however, who have the key to the lock, can slip out of this prison from time to time and see how the other half live. We also remember earlier experiences in earlier lives. I know it all seems a bit unlikely and, unless you've experienced it I can't really expect you to believe it. If it wasn't for the fact that in a few cases it can be used in healing situations I wouldn't even bother to mention it.

I had to think very carefully before adding this section to the book. After all credibility is something one builds up over a lifetime. A single false move and all one has worked for is lost. However I owe it to those who have had helpful reincarnation experiences to tell their stories because they might also help others. I also owe it to those who thought they had had a reincarnation experience only to discover later that it was nothing of the sort.

Being outside the body doesn't mean being in Heaven. That entails going into another dimension. It is much more difficult and only open to the spirit by invitation of a truly spiritual guide for special purposes. Once you are in the physical dimension that is where you stay until your allotted time is up. When a spirit frees itself of a body it is free of the electromagnetic forces which hold it to this planet or universe. By the power of thought it can be anywhere its thought waves have already reached. It happens to a lot of people but few like to admit it, probably because those of us who do admit to such truths are often open to abuse and ridicule from those who have no experience of such events.

One of the facts that becomes apparent, once your mind is open to receive wisdom, is that nothing is new. We have done it all before, and as the full extent of your own spiritual history becomes available to you it has a very sobering effect on the ego. Yes, I have a spiritual history of lives here and elsewhere and, in that, I am no different from anyone else. Reincarnation therapists use experiences of past lives to explain problems in this one. I rarely deliberately use healing to take people back beyond birth, though it has happened with clients in an ordinary healing situation.

PRE-BIRTH EXPERIENCES

So let us move slowly and carefully over this tricky area.

I'll start with the story of a woman whom I took back to a period before birth but after conception (while she was still in her mother's womb, in other words). This particular woman was terrified of cats (a phobia which goes by the even more terrifying name of ailurophobia, or gatophobia). She couldn't remember exactly when it had started, except that even as a child she couldn't bear to be near cats. When she went for a walk she took a dog with her to keep them away. So, in the usual way, I deactivated her logical consciousness and got straight into her subconscious. We went right through her childhood years, further and further back until birth. Even then it transpired that she was afraid of cats. Well there was only one thing for it I thought. We had to go into the pre-birth experience and there we found the cause of her problem.

Her mother had been terrified of cats and one day when she was about five to six months pregnant she had been surrounded by several of them in a friend's home. In panic she began to cry out, 'Get the cats away, get the cats away. They will kill my baby.' The strength of the emotion, the fear, was immediately imprinted on the unborn baby's mind. This was an emotional trauma experienced not only by the mother but conveyed to the memory banks of the unborn baby's subconscious. After that the child was to go through life with an unreasonable fear of cats.

Once she had experienced this past emotion as a healing therapy, she lost her fear of cats. She couldn't wait to go and find one, to pick it up and make up for all the years she had been terrified of them.

The next case also involves a pre-birth trauma. This woman lacked all sense of inner peace and had a feeling of terrible insecurity. On top of that she had an inferiority complex. She always felt that she was in the way, not worthy of attention and not really wanted or liked. But at the same time she needed people around her, and felt threatened if she was left on her own. She had a feeling of not being wanted, but a dread of doing anything about it — this woman really had a problem.

She easily regressed to a pre-birth situation in which she was able to recall clearly hearing her mother and father arguing. It appears that she had been an unwanted child and her father had tried to persuade her mother to have an abortion. Her mother, who also hadn't wanted the pregnancy, had thought about an abortion but been persuaded against it by the family doctor.

The woman clearly recalled the arguments for and against allowing her to be born. How can we even begin to imagine the anxiety that that must have caused the unborn infant, knowing that it was listening to an argument about its own life or death? The poor baby was in a 'no win' situation. If the argument for abortion won, its life would be taken before it had even begun. The spirit wouldn't die. After all, it's impossible to kill a spirit; all you do is deprive them of a life that they thought had become their own. But the feeling of rejection which that spirit experiences leaves a severe impression upon its mind which it carries forward into the next life.

Even if the argument goes in the baby's favour there will still be the feeling of not being wanted or loved, of being in the way, a feeling of guilt for having caused problems to the two parents. These feelings of insecurity, inferiority and guilt are carried forward into the world to affect the person's happiness and contentment throughout life. And because the subconscious so totally represses the memory of it all, the child and later the adult are unable to explain or deal with their emotional problems. I have had several cases like these. As parents we never realise how the word's we use in front of our children, born and unborn, can affect their future.

PAST LIFE EXPERIENCES

The following story involves a woman who suffered because her baby died due to problems in an earlier life. As I have already said I have thought very carefully about whether or not to include each of these cases. In every situation the overriding consideration has been, will the telling of this story help anyone? I know there are many who find the concept of reincarnation impossible to accept, while there are others who put every problem in this life down to difficulties experienced in a previous life. I have had so many experiences of clients going unexpectedly into past life situations that now I accept them without question. I am including this story simply because I believe it might help some parents who have lost a baby for no apparent reason, or whose baby may have suffered for months or years before passing away.

Jean came to me hoping I could cure her depression. She was in her early thirties and had been married about nine years. She had had a baby girl quite early on in her marriage and the baby had been born with a multitude of problems. Although the doctors had been wonderful the baby had suffered continual pain throughout its three-year life. Jean had not been able to have any more children and the loss of her only child, together with the suffering and pain it had had to endure before dying, had made Jean bitter and angry. She was full of resentment which she tried to conceal by taking a very demanding job, but eventually the memory of the tragic situation had become too much for her and depression had set in. All she initially told me was that she was suffering from depression. She didn't know why; she had no financial or health problems and she had a loyal, supportive husband.

As always in these situations I asked her to close her eyes while I put my hands over her head. This has the double effect of putting healing strength or energy into the patient, and allowing them to go deeper into their subconscious to find the real cause of the problem. Very quickly the healing love started releasing the hurt and Jean was in floods of tears. After a while she told me there was no God. 'How could a God', she asked, 'let a helpless little baby who couldn't possibly have hurt anyone suffer such terrible pain for three years?' She had prayed and gone to church, but there had been no help, no relief for her baby. No living God would allow this. 'I just can't believe in Him any more,' she said.

It was at this point that one of those rare but wonderful spiritual experiences happened. A presence filled the room. I don't have words to describe the emotions we experienced and witnessed. A feeling of great love, peace and well-being filled the entire room. Jean said afterwards that she would never again doubt the love and wisdom of God. It was an experience which would live with her for ever.

Still standing behind Jean I became aware of a story which

was vivid to both of us. I know that Jean also experienced the emotion of it, but whether she saw, heard and felt what I saw, heard and felt I cannot say, because this sort of spiritual experience is always very personal. The story Jean was given was this. Many years before, a lady had lived and enjoyed a peaceful and contented life and been fortunate enough to have several children, all of whom she had loved and cared for during her life. But when she was in her sixties cancer struck.

She was devastated. She had never been ill before and had always been the one to care for others. To be in a situation where others would have to care for her was something she couldn't get used to. She had believed that independence was a blessing and that dependence was a curse. She couldn't see that we need people who suffer just as much as we need those who care for them. How else can love grow except through the opportunity to give unselfishly to those who need?

We spend most of our lives learning to love by attending to others and the last few years of our life, as if to say thank you for the love we have been able to give, we ourselves become dependent on the caring love of others. But this woman couldn't understand this and, as the cancer got worse and it looked as if she would be unable to care for herself she took an overdose of drugs. She thought this would be better than becoming a burden upon her family. But by taking her own life she prevented others from learning how to love as she had learnt.

When she arrived back in the next world, where spiritual reality was made fully available to her, the horror of what she had done became apparent and she knew she would have to correct the wrong. She was given two choices. Relive a full life again to suffer those final years, or be born to suffer those final years immediately as a suffering child. She decided to suffer as a child and Jean, then still in the world of spirit and for reasons known only to her, agreed to come and live and give this woman the chance to be born as a suffering child. So Jean was born first. Eventually she married and had her baby, a baby destined to suffer and live for only three years. When the baby died it put right a previous wrong, and completed the purpose for which it had come.

Only those who have experienced a truly spiritual healing such as this can begin to understand the depth of its beauty and the enormous effect it has upon those who witness it. Jean's love returned in full, her depression lifted immediately, and she has been full of happiness ever since. There are many facets to healing, all of them beautiful.

Another reincarnation story is about a patient who had an unreasonable fear of getting on to boats. Her husband had bought one and was preparing to take it out for a few days' cruise. His wife became more and more nervous the closer the day of the expected voyage came. She was sure she would drown if she went to sea and thought this was some sort of premonition. She decided to come for treatment because her family had convinced her that it was just a phobia.

I gave her healing in the usual way. Straight away she began to tremble and it slowly got worse until her whole body was shaking violently. She was going through what is termed an 'abreaction'. This is the reliving of an emotion which has occurred earlier in life, usually during childhood. However it transpired that in the life before the present one she had drowned as a little girl. Somehow that emotional trauma had surfaced into this life. Relieved that it was just a past event and not a future one, she overcame her 'phobia' and has been to sea many times since then. Was it a past life experience? Who knows? The healing had the desired effect, and her fear of boats left her.

Apparent 'Past Life Experiences'

A week or two later Tony came to see me with his friend. He explained that he had a problem with which he needed help. Apparently he always went on the defensive if anyone started to ask him questions. If someone stopped him in the street and began to ask questions he would start to panic, feeling he was being interrogated. With his friend sitting just behind us, and Tony in the chair I use for healing, I proceeded in the usual way (that is, standing behind him with my hands over the top of his head). Almost immediately I got a reaction. And what a reaction, but not one I expected. Within a few minutes he started to stiffen until his body was solid and straight with his shoulders on the back of the chair and his backside resting on the edge of the front of the chair. His colour changed to a deep crimson, his tongue lolled out of the side of his mouth and his eyes popped until there was more white than pupil. For all the world he looked as if he had died.

I glanced at his friend who was quite obviously sure he had. I indicated that everything was under control and he mustn't panic. If anyone was going to panic I thought I had the right to be first. At that point his breathing also seemed to stop. I know it can't have been for more than a couple of minutes but, believe me, those two minutes seemed like hours. Never had I experienced anything like this.

Eventually he started to relax, his colour changed back from red to white, eyes and tongue were sucked back into their proper position and we all began to breathe again. I went and fetched him a glass of water, mainly as an excuse to have one myself. Within ten minutes he had totally recovered and was telling us how wonderful he was feeling. He said he felt confused. That seemed reasonable; so did I. He kept on about how fantastic he felt, how all his anger and fear just seemed to have left him and how he felt he had been enveloped in love.

He returned the following week and we were both convinced that he had had a past life experience. We thought he must have been hanged in a past life for some crime and this was why he didn't like facing people in interview situations. One reason for our thinking that it must have been a past life regression was that he would sometimes dream of a gallows and being locked in a dark room all alone. Whatever it was he was certainly a changed character. There were no inhibitions now. I thought that this was a satisfactory end to his problems.

But that wasn't the end of the story at all. He had to see me again some time later with an ordinary physical ailment and once again he quickly and easily went into the change-of-consciousness state. During this session it emerged that when he was a child he used to lie awake, frightened, looking out of his bedroom window which was the type with just four panes of glass. The cross-pieces of the wooden frames appeared to him as a scaffold and he used to lie there in his room alone and afraid. He was afraid of being asked certain questions by his father which his mother had told him not to speak of.

So there it was, nothing to do with a past life. But what about the abreaction, the stiff body, red face, popping eyes, lolling tongue? When he questioned his mother she told him that the umbilical cord had caught around his throat when he was born. The healing had actually released a birth trauma and the emotions of a little boy still scared to death of being questioned about things he now could no longer remember.

I have had many such experiences since that one. And whenever people come to me saying they can remember a past life I put it to the test of healing. Usually I find the cause in this life or just before birth. I have known people experience terrible emotions right through their lives, which when investigated in depth have turned out to be a father arguing with the pregnant mother and trying to persuade her to have an abortion.

At three months into pregnancy an unborn child is very aware of its parents' moods and feelings and takes particular interest in those discussions which involve its own well-being. The spirit which will become that child is prepared long before that for its life on earth. However, in spite of these views, I do believe in birth control which is essential to the well-being of those awaiting life. Now that science and technology have overcome disease and famine, which was nature's way of controlling a population, we must act to control the numbers ourselves or we will have done no more than replace one set of problems with another. But I am opposed to abortion as a method of birth control. So would you be if you had witnessed the fear that even talk of it can cause in the emotions of the unborn child. Where there is a genuine need for abortion such as a health risk, or a case of rape, then the rejected spirit will be able to accept the reasons behind the abortion.

——————— *PAST AND PRESENT LIVES* ———————

Why, I am often asked, if we have lived before do we have no recollection of it? This is because once we become one with the body and its perception, we have no choice but to utilise the body's system of communication and memory. This means that all memory of previous experience is lost to us, until we return.

The reason some people are able to remember flashes of previous lives, or be affected emotionally or physically by them, is that they either haven't become fully one with the physical at birth or some early shock or experience has affected the emotions in such a way that emotional consciousness is bypassed and spiritual perception is allowed through.

A lot of research has been done on this in America by renowned scientists and psychiatrists and most of the evidence points to reincarnation being fact. Obviously a lot more research is needed and many people will never be convinced, especially the very logically thinking who lack spiritual perception.

Each individual has to decide for themselves whether or not they believe in reincarnation. But there can be dangers in confusing events in our present lives with ones from previous lives. For example a woman came to me deeply distressed because she had remembered being sexually abused when she was a child. She had recalled all the details perfectly. The abuse had taken place when she was about five on a beautiful sunny day while walking across some grassy fields with one of her family.

When they came to the edge of the field the relative suggested that they sit down and the abuse took place. She had been able to remember every little detail and was convinced that she has been sexually abused as a child. However, after some searching questions and a session of regression therapy it turned out that what she had remembered were experiences from a previous life.

On the day she had recalled the incident she had been in a very relaxed (i.e. hypnotic) state. The situation was similar to the one she had found herself in when she was five in a previous life and the past memory had been able to filter through into her current thinking. We quickly sorted it out but it is very easy to see how emotionally sensitive individuals can cross the threshold between current and past experiences to cause chaos in a present life.

I have had people travel back across time and space to relive, or remember, many past lives. I don't as a rule encourage it, but if it happens naturally — as in the cases described above — I will see it through to the end. I have not yet had Napoleon, or a President, or a Pope. If I did I would have to find what inadequacies were present in this life because often when the mind cannot cope with current life problems it overcomes them by seeing them as part of a distant past life. In this way it avoids responsibility or fear in this life.

I know that it is supposed to take a little time and effort to induce the hypnotic state for regression, but I'm a healer not a hypnotist. I don't use any particular method. However if the client needs to know the cause of their present difficulties and the cause may lie in some distant past then I will help them to retrieve those details. I need to be absolutely sure of the need before agreeing to regression. And even then I will first try every other healing procedure I know to determine whether the desired supposed regression is a smokescreen to hide current insecurities. For those who have experienced OBE or regression there will be no doubts. For the rest of you I have no proof. And it really isn't important anyway, unless a tragedy in a previous life is causing problems in this one.

A woman well educated and with a good job, came asking if I would help with a phobia. For some inexplicable reason she just couldn't bring herself to go through a marriage ceremony. She had been engaged to be married but had kept putting the date back until eventually her fiancé lost patience and left.

It was a peculiar healing session in that not a lot seemed to be happening and then suddenly there we were, or rather there she was, supposedly back in some pre-life situation in which she had been a nun and a very pious one. As a nun she had of course been married to Jesus and so strong was this unconscious sense of commitment to Him that she couldn't go through a wedding ceremony in a church even in this life.

For once I forgot my own code of practice: 'Find the cause of the problem as quickly as possible and don't go into matters further than absolutely necessary.' I am there to heal people of their phobias or illness, not to satisfy their or my curiosity. However, for some reason, I just had to push further back. This was because she had said she had become a nun to avoid getting married. The thought of any physical relationship with a man had so appalled her that she had become a nun to avoid it.

Now this really made me curious. Why didn't she like men, or at least a physical relationship with them? So we went back further to the life before that one. In that life she had been a man, a very forceful, powerful man. So that was it. Being born a woman hadn't overcome the male feelings which had persisted from the previous life and which caused her to feel revolted at the thought of getting into bed with a man. To avoid it, she/he became a nun.

Perhaps the best example of how a past life experience can affect the present life is illustrated in the following story. I was phoned early one morning to ask if I would help someone who was very depressed. The history was a complex one. She had a deep feeling of being unwanted, lonely and of no value. For many years she had had a succession of illnesses, some quite serious. The woman was now in deep depression and had an overwhelming sense of loneliness and being unloved.

She arrived in the evening. I had set aside the whole evening because when I start to unravel the emotions of someone in depression I like to keep going until the cause and the answer have been found. Should a depressed person leave a consultation with their deeper emotions only partially released, it can in some instances put them into deeper crisis in the days following the consultation. I prefer, if possible, and it isn't always practical, to deal with those sort of problems in one session, even if it takes over an hour.

I sat the woman in a comfortable chair, went behind her and in the usual way put my hand over her head. Almost immediately she went into a relaxed state. Within minutes she was in floods of tears and for about ten minutes she wept as though her heart would break. Eventually, when she had got this emotion out of her system and was more in control of her thoughts, I asked her to remember what she was doing in her fourth year. She quickly remembered being on holiday. She didn't know where but she was with her family at an amusement fair. All seemed well until she noticed that she was alone. She had somehow become separated from the other members of the family. Panic struck, for search as she might they couldn't be found. From the emotions she exhibited this had obviously had a critical effect on her. Eventually a kindly stranger took her to the police and they found her parents for her. But still the overriding thoughts were those of loneliness and not being wanted.

Next I asked her to go back to the day she was born. All she could recall of that was feeling unwanted and very alone. So I asked her to go back to a pre-birth situation. What I was searching for was a time when she hadn't felt lonely and unloved so that we could move slowly forward from that point until we encountered the rejection. Even in the womb, though, she felt lonely and rejected. I wasn't making any progress so I decided to go even further back and into a pre-life situation. This was something I hadn't planned to do but I could see no alternative.

'I am going to count to three,' I told her. She was now in a hypnotised state though fully conscious and aware of all that was happening.

'On the count of three I want you to travel back to your previous life. I want you to be in your twentieth year of that life. One, Two, Three. You are now twenty. What are you doing?'

I hadn't chosen twenty for any particular reason other than that it seemed a good place to begin. Let's face it, if you aren't happy at twenty when will you be happy?

'I'm sitting under some trees,' she said.

'What's in front of you?'

'I don't know.'

'What is behind you?'

'Just trees.'

'How do you feel?' I asked.

'Very lonely, deserted, not wanted,' she answered.

This isn't getting me anywhere, I thought.

'When I count to three I want you to be five years old in the life you are experiencing.'

There was nothing else to do but keep regressing until I found a period when she was happy, even if it took all night and I was beginning to think it might.

'One. Two. Three. You are now five years old.' It was then that I got what I had been waiting for, a smile and then a chuckle.

'Is someone with you?'

'Yes.'

People in this state rarely volunteer information. You have to prise it out, a word at a time.

'Who is with you?'

'Other children.'

'Are your parents there?'

'I don't think so.'

'Can you see any grown up people?'

'No.'

'How many other children can you see?'

'I can't see any.'

'Are you blind?'

'Yes.'

So that was it. In the previous life she had been born blind. From this point I could begin to piece together her history to the present day.

'Are you in a children's home?'

'Yes.'

'When did you leave there?'

'When I was five, I think.'

'Where did you go?'

'To a farm.'

'Who looked after you?'

'Two people, husband and wife.'

'What did you do?'

'They sat me under the trees while they worked in the fields.'

So that was why she couldn't see anything when I questioned her earlier.

'How old were you when they died?'

'Twenty-two I think.'

'What did you do then?'

'I stayed in the house all the time.'

'For the rest of your life?'

'Yes.'

'How old were you when you died?'

'Eighty-five.'

'During those years you were alone, did you have any friends or a boy friend?'

'No. I was so very lonely.'

At this point I got a few more tears.

'When I count to three I want you to come forward to the day you were born in this life,' I said.

Now I had to find out what it was that had triggered the release of the past life's loneliness into this life's thoughts. I already knew that the panic of being lost when she was about four would have been one factor, but there had to be more to cause such depression later in life.

'One. Two. Three. You are now a baby of a few months old. How are you feeling?'

'Very lonely.'

'When do you feel loneliest?'

'At night. It's dark and I'm on my own.' (Tears again.) 'I want to be picked up. Nobody comes. I'm crying and getting cross. I'm lonely, it's dark. I want someone.'

'Why don't your parents come?'

'They don't want me, they don't love me.'

'Does anyone cuddle you?'

'Yes, Nanna does.'

'Are you happy with Nanna?'

'Yes, she holds me.'

'How old are you when Nanna dies?'

'I am twenty-two.'

I didn't know Nanna had died but now everything was fitting into place. I had found the cause of her depression. Now I had to effect a cure.

'How long ago was that?'

'Twelve years.'

'How do you feel now?'

'Now that Nanna has gone I feel lonely and lost again and unprotected. There's no one to look after me.'

That word 'again' said it all.

'But this time you have eyes, you can see, you don't need someone to look after you. This time you can be happy, free and look after others if you want to. When I count to five open your eyes and be free of the past and its loneliness.'

Well, that was it. We had a chat and she left an hour later with an explanation for twelve years of depression. Now she knew the cause she could do something about it.

For twelve years she had been in deep depression, feeling lonely and rejected. She had had all sorts of quite serious illnesses, which her subconscious had deliberately caused to attract attention, to get someone to care for her. As a baby she had been scared of the dark, felt insecure and lost or lonely in the dark. Remembering that she had had eighty-five years without sight and probably sixty or more of those on her own it's not surprising that the dark caused some unknown fear to trouble her.

Her grandmother, Nanna, was the one with the most time to spend with her. I wonder if the old people in the earlier life had been her grandparents? I wish now I had thought to ask. Her Nanna died when she was twenty-two, about the same age as when she lost the companionship of the old people in the previous life. Grief and shock at having lost Nanna would almost certainly have been enough to bring the loneliness of those earlier years to the surface. She would be experiencing all the emotions of those earlier times without knowing why.

Healing helped to lift her out of her grief; it also gave her an explanation for all those years of depression, and once all the emotions had been identified relative to the situation her depression lifted and another human being knew that she had experienced the miracle of healing.

Very often pains or other physical problems which have defied all attempts to cure them can have their origins in a past life.

One I recall clearly because it happened at a healing lecture which I was giving. A woman asked if I could help with a pain she had had in her left knee since she was about nine. I guessed that she was now about forty. The pain, which was constant, had no apparent cause. She had received all the usual conventional treatment and also a lot of unconventional treatment as well. She came to the front of the room. I asked her to stand facing the audience with her eyes closed. I placed my hand over her head which had the immediate effect of bringing her subconscious to the surface. She began swaying around and declared that she could see herself riding a horse. She could see she was wearing some sort of red uniform. It was then she realised that she was a soldier riding into battle in some previous life. Still with her eyes closed and swaying, quite uncontrollably, she told how her horse was shot from under her. At this point she collapsed to the floor onto her left side. She immediately began to feel distressed and cried out that the horse had fallen onto her left leg and that she was trapped. She told how the horse struggled and fell across her chest. She then went very quiet for a few moments before telling us how she was now free of her body and in a beautiful, peaceful place. She was being directed towards a brilliant white light which she knew was 'the way home'.

At this point I released her from the healing power and she returned to full logical awareness. She got up and told the audience how she hadn't wanted to return to her body because of the peace and beauty she had found. This is a very common expression of those who have experienced dying in a past life. More importantly the pain in her knee had gone and it has never returned. This case is not exceptional, I have seen many 'mysterious symptoms' disappear after the patient has been through a reincarnation therapy to discover the cause.

Before moving away from this subject, I want to make a very important point about using reincarnation therapy to help cure current anxiety or other health problems. It is this: the subconscious *can* lie. If you take everything which comes out of a deeply relaxed (i.e. hypnotised) person as factual, you will be creating new and bigger problems both for yourself and those you are trying to help. When dealing with the memories released by the subconscious either in the mildly relaxed or deeply relaxed state it is essential to interpret them correctly.

Here is a case in point. A woman came to me who had suffered depression for many years and who also had a fear of being questioned. Whenever she was questioned she would always answer, 'I don't know,' even when she did know the answer. We went through the usual routine of trying to find the problem in her early years but to no avail. So I took her back into her previous life. She quickly remembered being interrogated, in a small room, a cell she was sure. She recalled that the questioning, or rather interrogation, was brutal, with threats of what would happen to her if she didn't answer.

She believed herself in that life to be about eighteen. She also recalled that she was being interrogated by the Inquisition and that one priest in particular was very threatening. After several sessions it emerged that she was a novice nun who had had an affair with a young priest and the order to which she belonged had found out. What they did not know was which priest it was who had sinned against her. In order to protect this priest she answered every question with 'I don't know.' There was no doubt in her mind that she had experienced a past life under hypnosis.

However I'm afraid I never totally trust what the subconscious tells me and something just did not seem right, especially as her anxieties had not lessened. So, after three or four of these regression sessions, I went back to ordinary healing, without any warning. This had the effect of creating confusion. The subconscious was all prepared to regress back to a previous life, but I stopped it short and kept it in this one. Now a totally different story emerged.

As a young girl she had had an affair with an older boy. Her father had found out and put her through a very searching interrogation. Of course she felt guilty and ashamed, and it was this guilt which had prevented her from releasing the story originally. Moving the whole incident into a previous life absolved her of responsibility for what had occurred so that she could discuss it.

'Why the priest and Inquisition?' I hear you ask. Another word for priest is 'Father'. At the time she was a virgin, or had been until the incident with the older boy; a nun is a virgin. And so we have all the factors necessary for a very convincing deception. The woman involved had no conscious intention of misleading me. Her sole reason for seeking help was to find out the truth about her anxieties. She totally believed what her subconscious wanted her to believe. The subconscious had been doing its job of protecting her against what it thought would be further trauma.

In all cases of trauma release you must be sure to use only qualified therapists who belong to nationally recognised organisations and who have experience of interpreting the words, emotions and actions of your subconscious. To believe literally what you think you remember may be self-delusion.

Epilogue

Healing is an art once practised by doctors who, using their academic skills, knowledge of the patient and his circumstances and a high degree of intuition, could often prevent many illnesses from becoming serious or needing more specialist treatment. In fact doctors of earlier generations were more than local GPs. They were also local healers. But that was in the days of the 'family doctor' who had time to sit and listen.

That time is no longer available to most doctors and, because of advances in chemical and technological forms of treatment which are beyond the means of most local GPs to administer, they are finding that more and more frequently they need to refer their patients to the specialist. There is a great danger that the GP will eventually become no more than a local chemist and a clearing house for hospitals. The GP's role will be merely to decide which specialist a patient should be referred to, after a course of locally prescribed drugs has not cured the problem. This is not the doctor's fault. Once the patient moves beyond his local GP to have his symptoms considered by a specialist consultant, any thought of healing the whole person is lost.

Over the last fifty years or so, care and treatment of the sick has become more specialised, with each discipline isolating itself and not interfering in those areas of health which it considers belong to some other department. Health care should not be about this bit or that bit; it is very much about the interaction between body, mind and spirit — machine, computer and driver. Health will always be greater than just the sum of its parts. It is about life, and this is beyond technology to fathom.

Because of dissatisfaction with drug therapy which treats the symptoms, but often not the cause, more and more people are turning to alternative forms of treatment: treatments which look at the relationship between body and mind and try to use one to help the other. The practitioners of alternative and complementary medicine are now beginning to do the job that was once thought to be the exclusive domain of the GP.

Alternative and complementary therapists realise the importance of the relationship between themselves and patients. They know that without confidence in the therapist there can be no cure, no healing. But trust and confidence don't just happen; they have to be built into a relationship. Reputation alone is not sufficient. Every patient has to be considered individually.

Unfortunately the credibility of our doctors is declining fast. They are no longer considered infallible and those who do try to care for their patients often don't have the necessary time to spend listening to them. Patients need to feel that those they trust with their health will care about it, and consider it carefully. They need to know that the doctor will have sufficient time, authority, ability and trust in his own judgement so that there will be no need to question the treatment offered, that he will follow their progress right through. This happens less and less. And so the public have begun to look elsewhere for counselling, with the result that anyone who feels the need to help another can join one of the growing army of alternative practitioners who, after some introductory instruction, become responsible for the health and emotions of other human beings.

This may or may not be the best way to proceed, but it does show that people prefer time and consideration to drugs and medical technology. The number of different alternative health treatments on offer to the public grows each year. They flourish in a country where the care of the nation's health is supposed to be one of the most advanced in the world and this is a direct indictment of the authorities who decide which direction the health industry should take.

The miracle of healing is beyond a doctor's science. Doctors don't heal; they cut, carve, remove, poison or burn to rid the body of that which ails it. But when they sew the pieces back together again they know that a force beyond their understanding does the healing. With their supreme understanding of medical science and their technological skills, doctors must still — in the final analysis — put their faith in a factor beyond science and technology and trust that this unknown force will take over and heal the patient when their work is done.

Doctors apply their skills to quantifiable science; healers apply their skills to the unquantifiable forces of life. There is no need for acrimony between the two groups. The public need both, and each needs to have a basic understanding of the work of the other. The hospital doctor's primary interest in his patient has become biological. He sees the patient as a unit and personal involvement is kept to a minimum. Sadly, this is becoming the case with many family doctors.

A healer's interest in his patient is to understand him as an individual and use his gift to give him extra strength or vitality so that the patient's own life-force, his spirit, can take advantage of what the doctor's technology is doing for him — though that technology often wouldn't be necessary if the patient could recognise the power within himself.

However, as long as healers persist in believing that because healing is a gift no further effort is necessary to improve or influence that gift, they will remain as amateurs outside the mainstream of health care. It is true that healing is a gift; but it is arrant nonsense for healers to suggest that they don't need to provide proof of minimum standards of excellence before declaring themselves proficient in the art of caring for the welfare of others.

Artists have a gift, surgeons have a gift, stockmen have a gift.

Epilogue

I was taught that stockmen are born, not made, and the same is true of healers. However all the great artists received training and tuition; fortunately so do surgeons; and no horse-trainer would put his horses into the care of a stockman who hadn't received training, no matter how superior his gift.

Healers also need training and education to fully develop, use, and understand their gifts. Basic instruction in counselling, psychotherapy, physiology, biology, religions, metaphysics and any other subject directly or indirectly involved with their work is a necessity if healers are going to forward their cause. It is true a mother doesn't need a certificate or diploma to love and care for her children, but she does if she is going to be responsible for other people's children as a teacher, counsellor, etc.

When healers begin to take themselves seriously, so will the medical profession. Healing therapy is desperately needed to cure the causes of many of the nation's health problems because drug therapy is not the whole answer. I believe that the medical profession has lost its way in a jungle of medical technology. It has been reduced to treating symptoms which the subconscious will go on producing irrespective of medical treatment until someone goes beyond the symptoms and identifies the cause. This is true healing.

Resources

Bibliography

This book involved a limited use of reference material because it is largely the result of personal experience. However two books have been of particular value to the author and they are listed here so that others may make use of the information they contain.

Robert D. Becker, MD, and Gary Seldon, *The Body Electric*, Quill, William Morrow, New York, 1985.

Dr Wayne W. Dyer, *Your Erroneous Zones*, Sphere Books Ltd, London, 1976.

Useful Addresses

For further information on healing contact:

National Federation of Spiritual Healers (NFSH),
Old Manor Farm Studio, Church Street, Sunbury-on-Thames, Middlesex TW16 6RG

Index

Index